Hematology and Oncology Pearls

Hematology and Oncology Pearls

MICHAEL A. DANSO, MD
Chief Fellow
Medical Oncology and Hematology Service
Memorial Sloan-Kettering Cancer Center
New York, New York

ETHAN M. BASCH, MD
Fellow
Medical Oncology and Hematology Service
Memorial Sloan-Kettering Cancer Center
New York, New York

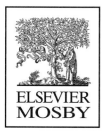

ELSEVIER
MOSBY

The Curtis Center
170 S Independence Mall W 300E
Philadelphia, Pennsylvania 19106

Hematology and Oncology Pearls   ISBN: 1-56053-577-6

NOTICE

Medicine is an ever-changing field. Standard safety precautions must be followed, but as new research and clinical experience broaden our knowledge, changes in treatment and drug therapy may become necessary or appropriate. Readers are advised to check the most current product information provided by the manufacturer of each drug to be administered to verify the recommended dose, the method and duration of administration, and contraindications. It is the responsibility of the licensed prescriber, relying on experience and knowledge of the patient, to determine dosages and the best treatment for each individual patient. Neither the publisher nor the author assumes any liability for any injury and/or damage to persons or property arising from this publication.

Library of Congress Cataloging-in-Publication Data
Hematology and oncology pearls / editors, Michael Danso, Ethan Basch.—1st ed.
  p. ; cm.—(The Pearls series)
 Includes index.
 ISBN 1-56053-577-6
 1. Cancer—Case studies. 2. Blood—Diseases—Case studies. I. Danso, Michael. II. Basch, Ethan M. III. Series.
  [DNLM: 1. Hematologic Diseases—diagnosis. 2. Neoplasms—diagnosis. WH 120 H4867 2005]
RC262.H445 2005
616.99418—dc22
                                                                                2005041490

Acquisitions Editor: Linda Belfus
Developmental Editor: Jacqueline Mahon
Project Manager: Cecelia Bayruns

Working together to grow
libraries in developing countries

www.elsevier.com | www.bookaid.org | www.sabre.org

ELSEVIER   BOOK AID International   Sabre Foundation

Printed in the United States of America.

Last digit is the print number: 9 8 7 6 5 4 3 2 1

CONTENTS

CONTRIBUTORS

Ethan M. Basch, MD
Fellow, Medical Oncology and Hematology Service, Memorial Sloan-Kettering Cancer Center, New York, New York

Kathleen Beekman, MD
Chief Fellow, Medical Oncology and Hematology Service, Memorial Sloan-Kettering Cancer Center, New York, New York

Emily Chan, MD, PhD
Fellow, Medical Oncology and Hematology Service, Memorial Sloan-Kettering Cancer Center, New York, New York

Anne Chiang, MD, PhD
Fellow, Medical Oncology and Hematology Service, Memorial Sloan-Kettering Cancer Center, New York, New York

Adam Cohen, MD
Fellow, Medical Oncology and Hematology Service, Memorial Sloan-Kettering Cancer Center, New York, New York

Michael A. Danso, MD
Chief Fellow, Medical Oncology and Hematology Service, Memorial Sloan-Kettering Cancer Center, New York, New York

Leslie Ellis, MD
Fellow, Medical Oncology and Hematology Service, Memorial Sloan-Kettering Cancer Center, New York, New York

David Feltquate, MD, PhD
Fellow, Medical Oncology and Hematology Service, Memorial Sloan-Kettering Cancer Center, New York, New York

Mark Fleming, MD
Fellow, Medical Oncology and Hematology Service, Memorial Sloan-Kettering Cancer Center, New York, New York

Matthew Fury, MD, PhD
Fellow, Medical Oncology and Hematology Service, Memorial Sloan-Kettering Cancer Center, New York, New York

Matthew Galsky, MD
Clinical Assistant Physician, Medical Oncology and Hematology Service, Memorial Sloan-Kettering Cancer Center, New York, New York

John Gerecitano, MD, PhD
Fellow, Medical Oncology and Hematology Service, Memorial Sloan-Kettering Cancer Center, New York, New York

Jeffrey Halaas, MD, PhD
Fellow, Medical Oncology and Hematology Service, Memorial Sloan-Kettering Cancer Center, New York, New York

Gregory Leonard, MD
Fellow, Gastrointestinal Oncology Service, Memorial Sloan-Kettering Cancer Center, New York, New York

Michaela Liedtke, MD
Fellow, Medical Oncology and Hematology Service, Memorial Sloan-Kettering Cancer Center, New York, New York

Igor Matushansky, MD
Fellow, Medical Oncology and Hematology Service, Memorial Sloan-Kettering Cancer Center, New York, New York

Daniel Milton, MD
Fellow, Medical Oncology and Hematology Service, Memorial Sloan-Kettering Cancer Center, New York, New York

Luke Nordquist, MD
Fellow, Medical Oncology and Hematology Service, Memorial Sloan-Kettering Cancer Center, New York, New York

Daniel Persky, MD
Fellow, Medical Oncology and Hematology Service, Memorial Sloan-Kettering Cancer Center, New York, New York

Carlos Ramos, MD
Fellow, Medical Oncology and Hematology Service, Memorial Sloan-Kettering Cancer Center, New York, New York

Gregory Riely, MD, PhD
Chief Fellow, Medical Oncology and Hematology Service, Memorial Sloan-Kettering Cancer Center, New York, New York

Petra Rietschel, MD, PhD
Fellow, Medical Oncology and Hematology Service, Memorial Sloan-Kettering Cancer Center, New York, New York

Ellen Ronnen, MD
Fellow, Medical Oncology and Hematology Service, Memorial Sloan-Kettering Cancer Center, New York, New York

Karen Smith, MD, MPH
Fellow, Medical Oncology and Hematology Service, Memorial Sloan-Kettering Cancer Center, New York, New York

Mika A. Sovak, MD, PhD
Fellow, Medical Oncology and Hematology Service, Memorial Sloan-Kettering Cancer Center, New York, New York

Yungpo Bernard Su, MD
Clinical Assistant Physician, Medical Oncology Service, Memorial Sloan-Kettering Cancer Center, New York, New York

Tiffany Traina, MD
Chief Fellow, Medical Oncology and Hematology Service, Memorial Sloan-Kettering Cancer Center, New York, New York

Jennifer Wheler, MD
Fellow, Medical Oncology and Hematology Service, Memorial Sloan-Kettering Cancer Center, New York, New York

FOREWORD

The field of medical oncology has seen extraordinary recent advances in our knowledge of disease mechanisms, development of novel therapies, and understanding of the patient experience. Modern medical oncologists face the challenge of keeping up with this rapidly evolving field.

This text, written by fellows and reviewed by faculty at Memorial Sloan-Kettering Cancer Center, represents a commitment to patient care informed by scholarship and research. The editors have selected clinical scenarios to assist the reader in understanding clinical decision making, calling upon the best available scientific evidence, current standards of care, and sensitivity to the needs of the patient. Synthesis of clinical trial data is provided to orient the reader to the current state of research for each discussed type of cancer and stage, with an eye to future developments.

The fellowship program at Memorial Sloan-Kettering Cancer Center provides trainees and young investigators with a deep yet flexible framework for the application of knowledge, the background necessary to recognize the unusual, and the inspiration to address unresolved research questions based on problems recognized at the bedside. It is our hope that the reader of this compendium will capture some of this spirit as well.

GEORGE J. BOSL, MD
CHAIRMAN, DEPARTMENT OF MEDICINE
PATRICK M. BYRNE CHAIR IN CLINICAL ONCOLOGY
MEMORIAL SLOAN-KETTERING CANCER CENTER
NEW YORK, NEW YORK

PREFACE

We are pleased to introduce the first edition of *Hematology and Oncology Pearls*, a collaborative effort of fellows and faculty in the Hematology and Oncology Services at Memorial Sloan-Kettering Cancer Center. The included cases are designed to provide current teaching in both common and unusual clinical scenarios referred to the hematologist and oncologist. The text is in part inspired by our weekly "post clinic conference"—a popular case-based educational consortium—where challenging cases are presented by fellows to select faculty for discussion.

Although many excellent reference texts exist in the fields of hematology and oncology, this book offers a unique case-based format that stimulates the reader to consider a differential diagnosis and management plan. As a reflection of the patients who are commonly referred to Memorial Sloan-Kettering Cancer Center, our explorations here are weighted towards malignant hematology and solid tumor oncology. This book also provides a review of the common malignancies that a practicing medical oncologist is likely to encounter.

Our intention is to provide a valuable resource for medical students, residents, and generalists with an interest in hematology and oncology. Fellows in hematology/oncology training programs will find the format useful not only for preparation for board examinations but also as an important evidence-based compendium for clinics. Similarly, the practicing hematology/oncology specialist may find many of the cases presented both interesting and challenging.

MICHAEL A. DANSO, MD
ETHAN M. BASCH, MD
EDITORS

ACKNOWLEDGMENTS

This text represents the cumulative efforts of more than 50 medical oncology fellows and faculty members at Memorial Sloan-Kettering Cancer Center. Meticulous work and research by each contributor has yielded a book that we hope will be useful to readers. Our aim is to inspire the same sense of enthusiasm, compassion, and scientific curiosity as embodied by its many authors.

We respectfully acknowledge those patients whose cases are presented herein; it is to their health and memories that we dedicate these pages. The fellowship program is particularly grateful to those faculty members and mentors who generously give their time to our educations and who have provided guidance and editorial review of these chapters.

The academic context and collaborative spirit at Memorial Sloan-Kettering have provided an ideal environment for this effort. In particular, we would like to thank our fellowship director, Dean Bajorin, who has provided enormous encouragement and support of our professional development as medical oncologists and who has served as a strong advocate of this project. George Bosl, Chairman of Medicine, is an incomparable scholar whose love of this field and of knowledge has inspired generations of housestaff, including the contributors to this volume.

Administrative support from the Office of Education and Training has been invaluable, particularly from Cheryl James, Liana Purnama, and Lillie Dilaurao. Finally, we would like to thank our friends and families for their support and understanding, particularly Elizabeth.

REVIEWERS

We are indebted to the following Attending Physicians for reviewing the cases presented.

Breast Oncology Service

Maura Dickler, MD
Assistant Attending Physician, Memorial Sloan-Kettering Cancer Center

Clifford Hudis, MD
Chief, Breast Cancer Medicine Service, Memorial Sloan-Kettering Cancer Center

Andrew Seidman, MD
Associate Attending Physician, Memorial Sloan-Kettering Cancer Center

Genitourinary Oncology Service

George J. Bosl, MD
Chairman, Department of Medicine
Attending Physician, Memorial Sloan-Kettering Cancer Center

Dean F. Bajorin, MD, FACP
Program Director, Medical Oncology, Hematology Fellowship
Attending Physician, Memorial Sloan-Kettering Cancer Center

Beverly Drucker, MD
Clinical Assistant Physician, Memorial Sloan-Kettering Cancer Center

Lewis Kampel, MD
Associate Attending Physician, Memorial Sloan-Kettering Cancer Center

Michael J. Morris, MD
Clinical Assistant Physician, Memorial Sloan-Kettering Cancer Center

Susan F. Slovin, MD, PhD
Assistant Attending Physician, Memorial Sloan-Kettering Cancer Center

Gastrointestinal Oncology Service

Ghassan K. Abou-Alfa, MD
Clinical Assistant Physician, Memorial Sloan-Kettering Cancer Center

David H. Ilson, MD, PhD
Associate Attending Physician, Memorial Sloan-Kettering Cancer Center

Nancy E. Kemeny, MD
Attending Physician, Memorial Sloan-Kettering Cancer Center

Jeremy S. Kortmansky, MD
Clinical Assistant Physician, Memorial Sloan-Kettering Cancer Center

Robert G. Maki, MD, PhD
Assistant Attending Physician, Memorial Sloan-Kettering Cancer Center

Eileen M. O'Reilly, MBBCh, BAO
Assistant Attending Physician, Memorial Sloan-Kettering Cancer Center

Leonard B. Saltz, MD
Attending Physician, Memorial Sloan-Kettering Cancer Center

Deborah Schrag, MD, MPH
Assistant Attending Physician, Memorial Sloan-Kettering Cancer Center

Manish A. Shah, MD
Clinical Assistant Physician, Memorial Sloan-Kettering Cancer Center

Thoracic Oncology Service

Christopher G. Azzoli, MD
Clinical Assistant Physician, Memorial Sloan-Kettering Cancer Center

Lee M. Krug, MD
Assistant Attending Physician, Memorial Sloan-Kettering Cancer Center

Vincent A. Miller, MD
Assistant Attending Physician, Memorial Sloan-Kettering Cancer Center

Head and Neck Oncology Service

David G. Pfister, MD
Attending Physician, Memorial Sloan-Kettering Cancer Center

Immunology Service

Wen-Jen Hwu, MD, PhD
Assistant Attending Physician, Memorial Sloan-Kettering Cancer Center

Jedd D. Wolchok, MD, PhD
Assistant Attending Physician, Memorial Sloan-Kettering Cancer Center

Leukemia Service

Mark L. Heaney, MD, PhD
Co-Director, Medical Oncology/Hematology Fellowship Program
Assistant Attending Physician, Memorial Sloan-Kettering Cancer Center

Lymphoma Service

Paul A. Hamlin, MD
Clinical Assistant Physician, Memorial Sloan-Kettering Cancer Center

Steve M. Horowitz, MD
Clinical Assistant Physician, Memorial Sloan-Kettering Cancer Center

Carol S. Portlock, MD
Attending Physician, Memorial Sloan-Kettering Cancer Center

Gynecology-Oncology Service

Carol Aghajanian, MD
Assistant Attending Physician, Memorial Sloan-Kettering Cancer Center

Jakob Dupont, MD
Clinical Assistant Physician, Memorial Sloan-Kettering Cancer Center

Hematology Service

Raymond L. Comenzo, MD
Associate Attending Physician, Memorial Sloan-Kettering Cancer Center

Hani Hassoun, MD
Associate Attending Physician, Memorial Sloan-Kettering Cancer Center

Allogenic Transplant Service

Esperanza B. Papadopoulos, MD
Associate Attending Physician, Memorial Sloan-Kettering Cancer Center

PATIENT 1

A 45-year-old man with a pathological fracture of the right femur

A 45-year-old man with no significant medical history is admitted to the hospital after suffering a fracture of his right proximal femur. Review of symptoms is positive for mild shortness of breath on exertion and an ache in his right thigh, intermittently for 2 months. He smokes two packs of cigarettes a day and has done so for 30 years.

Physical Examination: Temperature 36.6°C, blood pressure 160/90 mmHg, pulse 110. General: well-nourished. HEENT: mild pallor, anicteric, no adenopathy. Cardiovascular: regular rate and rhythm without murmurs. Chest: clear to auscultation. Abdomen: palpable spleen tip, no hepatomegaly, no ascites. Extremities: right leg held in traction.

Laboratory Findings: Hemoglobin 10.1 g/dL, platelets 92,000/μL, WBC 24,200/μL (15% neutrophils, 1% bands, 16% lymphocytes, 26% plasma lymphocytes, 30% plasma cells). Liver function tests: normal. Chest radiograph: normal. Radiograph of right femur: lytic lesion at right proximal femur with nondisplaced fracture (see Figure).

Questions: What is the most likely diagnosis? What additional tests would you request to confirm this diagnosis?

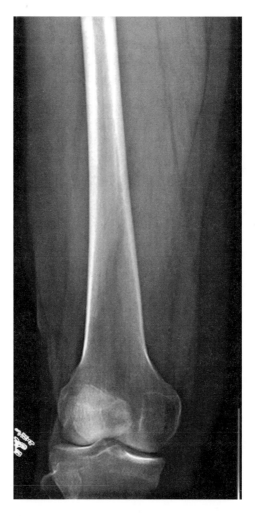

Answers: Plasma cell leukemia with osteolytic bone lesion is the likely conclusion. Several additional tests should be ordered, including lactate dehydrogenase (LDH), serum calcium, and serum protein electrophoresis.

Discussion: Plasma cell leukemia (PCL) is a rare variant of multiple myeloma and is defined by more than 2000/µL circulating plasma cells, or by the presence of more than 20% plasma cells, in the peripheral blood. PCL represents 2 to 4% of all myelomas. There are two recognized variants of PCL: Primary PCL is defined as a malignant plasma cell proliferation first diagnosed in the leukemic phase; the second form consists of a leukemic transformation in a previously diagnosed multiple myeloma. It represents a terminal event in patients with relapsed or refractory myeloma. Approximately 60% of PCLs are primary.

The median age at presentation is between 53 and 57 years, about 10 years younger than the median age at presentation with myeloma. PCL typically has a more aggressive clinical presentation than multiple myeloma, with a higher frequency of anemia, thrombocytopenia, hypercalcemia, renal impairment, and extramedullary involvement. The incidence of other poor prognostic indicators, such as a high LDH level, elevated β_2-microglobulin, and the proportion of S-phase plasma cells, are also higher in PCL.

There are several immunophenotypic distinctions between myeloma and PCL. In most case series, plasma cells from PCL consistently demonstrate a higher expression of CD20 antigen than cells from patients with myeloma, suggesting a more immature phenotype. The PCL cells also tend to lack CD56, which is thought to be an important antigen in anchoring plasma cells to bone marrow stroma. CD56 expression in myeloma has been associated with a better prognosis. CD28 positivity is also found more frequently in patients with primary PCL.

DNA hyperdiploidy is more common in multiple myeloma. In contrast, most patients with PCL have a diploid or hypodiploid cell content. Cytogenetic analysis demonstrates a high incidence of chromosome 13 monosomies in PCL in contrast to the low incidence found in myeloma. In myeloma this chromosomal abnormality is associated with a poor prognosis. Other cytogenetic findings that are associated with a favorable outcome in myeloma, such as trisomies of chromosomes 6, 9, and 17, are typically absent in primary PCL.

Additional investigations to request in the present patient should include a full biochemistry profile, LDH, serum calcium, serum protein electrophoresis, serum immunoelectrophoresis, urine protein electrophoresis, and β_2-microglobulin. A full skeletal survey should also be performed to look for additional lytic lesions. A CT scan of the abdomen to ascertain extramedullary involvement is also warranted.

With the multiple poor prognostic features present at diagnosis, it is not surprising that response to therapy in PCL is poor. The overall response rate ranges from 37 to 47%, with a median survival of 6.8 to 12 months. The response rate and survival are particularly poor in patients treated with melphalan and prednisone as compared to those given intensive combination chemotherapy. Typical combination chemotherapy is vincristine-Adriamycin-dexamethasone (VAD). Patients treated with combination chemotherapy may have response rates as high as 60%, with a median survival of 20 months. Given the poor prognosis of primary PCL, intensification with high-dose therapy, followed by stem cell rescue, should also be offered to patients. Patients with secondary PCL have a particularly poor outcome, with a median survival of 1 month.

In the present patient, mottling of the intermedullary right femur, consistent with myelomatous involvement, was evident on X-ray. He was treated with a cycle of VAD chemotherapy but responded poorly and had a rapidly progressive course. The patient died from complications of a respiratory tract infection within 8 weeks of diagnosis.

Clinical Pearls

1. PCL is a rare variant of multiple myeloma characterized by the presence of more than 2000/µL of circulating plasma cells or more than 20% plasma cells in the peripheral blood.

2. Primary PCL is defined as a malignant plasma cell proliferation first diagnosed in the leukemic phase. Secondary PCL consists of a leukemic transformation in a previously diagnosed multiple myeloma.

3. PCL has typically a more aggressive clinical presentation and a significantly worse prognosis than multiple myeloma.

4. Patients with PCL should be treated with combination chemotherapy.

REFERENCES

1. Blade J, Kyle RA: Nonsecretory myeloma, immunoglobulin D myeloma, and plasma cell leukemia. Hematol Oncol Clin North Am 13(6):1259-1271, 1999.
2. Garcia-Sanz R, Orfao A, Gonzalez M, et al: Primary plasma cell leukemia: Clinical, immunophenotypic, DNA ploidy, and cytogenetic characteristics. Blood 93(3):1032-1037, 1999.
3. Costello R, Sainty D, Bouabdallah R, et al: Primary plasma cell leukemia: A report of 18 cases. Leuk Res 25:103-107, 2001.

PATIENT 2

A 28-year-old man with a rapidly growing axillary mass

A 28-year-old man first noticed a small nodule in his left axilla 2 weeks prior to admission. During the next 10 days, the mass grew in size and was demonstrated on a computed tomography (CT) scan to be a conglomerate nodal mass, 7 cm in maximal diameter. Four days later, upon resection, it measured 11 cm. Pathological examination revealed intermediate-sized lymphocytes with interspersed pale phagocytic macrophages and a high proliferative index. Immunohistochemistry revealed the lymphocytes to be CD5(−), CD10(+), CD20(+), BCL2(−), with an MIB-1 greater than 95%.

Physical Examination: General: well-appearing. Vital signs: temperature 37.6°C, pulse 96, blood pressure 106/50 mmHg. HEENT: sclera anicteric. Lymph nodes: bulky adenopathy in left axilla; no cervical, supraclavicular, or inguinal lymphadenopathy. Cardiovascular: regular rate and rhythm without murmurs. Chest: clear to auscultation bilaterally. Abdomen: soft, nontender, nondistended. Extremities: no edema.

Laboratory Findings: CBC: hemoglobin 16.6 g/dL, WBC 8500/μL, platelets 285,000/μL. Biochemistry profile: potassium 4.4, BUN 15 mg/dL, creatinine 1.2 mg/dL, uric acid 4.2, LDH 660. Lymph node biopsy: monotonous intermediate-sized lymphocytes interspersed with macrophages in a "starry sky" pattern (see Figure).

Questions: What are the diagnosis and treatment plan? What is the most immediate risk when treatment is started for this patient?

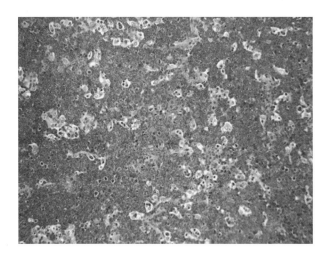

Answers: The diagnosis is Burkitt's lymphoma, stage IIA, high risk. Treatment should include aggressive combination chemotherapy, which carries a risk of tumor lysis syndrome.

Discussion: Burkitt's lymphoma (BL) is a highly aggressive B-cell lymphoma that accounts for 30% of nonendemic pediatric lymphomas but less than 1% of adult non-Hodgkin's lymphomas. Clonal expansion occurs when the c-myc onco-gene is overexpressed due to a translocation event that places it in proximity to a strong promoter, such as the Ig heavy chain locus. Cells with this translocation divide continuously, causing a tumor doubling time measured in hours. Diagnosis of BL is usually obvious, based on the history of a rapidly expansile mass and the pathological find-ing of monotonous medium-sized B-cells with a proliferative index greater than 99%. Unlike this patient, most sporadic cases present with intraab-dominal masses arising in the terminal ileum, cecum, or mesentery. Endemic cases present usu-ally as masses in the jaws or other facial bones.

Although rapidly fatal without treatment, BL is highly responsive to chemotherapy. Relapsed dis-ease is almost universally fatal, highlighting the importance of an aggressive initial approach. The CODOX-M/IVAC regimen developed at the National Cancer Institute has been shown to be curative in the majority of patients. This is an alternating non–cross-resistant regimen consist-ing of treatment with cyclophosphamide, vin-cristine, and doxorubicin, followed by a continuous infusion of high-dose methotrexate and consoli-dation with ifosfamide, etoposide, and cytarabine. Prophylactic intrathecal cytarabine and methotrex-ate are necessary to prevent relapse of disease in the central nervous system (CNS). High-risk patients (defined by elevated LDH, decreased performance status, high stage, and tumor mass greater than 10 cm) are treated with four cycles of alternating CODOX-M and IVAC, whereas low-risk patients (with none of the previously men-tioned risk factors) are treated with three cycles of CODOX-M alone. As in this case, the large major-ity of BL patients present with high-risk disease.

Because of the high tumor burden and rapid response to chemotherapy, tumor lysis is rapid and must be anticipated. Tumor lysis syndrome occurs when intracellular contents are released into the circulation, acutely increasing the con-centration of potassium, uric acid, and phospho-rus. Hyperkalemia can lead to dangerous cardiac arrhythmias, and uric acid and calcium phosphate can precipitate in the peripheral tissues and kid-neys, leading to acute renal failure. Prior to treat-ment, all BL patients should be started on prophylactic allopurinol and aggressive hydration to prevent these complications. Serum levels of uric acid, potassium, and phosphorus should be monitored frequently. Patients with larger tumor burdens and high LDH levels are at increased risk, and some will require hemodialysis for excessive hyperkalemia.

The present patient was successfully treated with CODOX-M/IVAC chemotherapy and is in complete clinical remission.

Clinical Pearls

1. Burkitt's lymphoma (BL) is a highly aggressive B-cell lymphoma that presents with rapidly growing lymphadenopathy (often in the abdomen).

2. BL is fatal without treatment but highly responsive to aggressive combination chemotherapy. Relapsed disease is almost universally fatal.

3. Patients are classified as high risk (elevated LDH, decreased performance status, high stage, tumor mass greater than 10 cm) or low risk (absence of these characteris-tics). The approach to treatment varies according to risk category.

4. CNS involvement is common, and intrathecal prophylaxis is mandatory.

5. Tumor lysis syndrome is common during treatment for BL, particularly in patients with high tumor burden and/or elevated baseline LDH levels. Potassium, uric acid, and phosphorus levels should be monitored closely.

REFERENCES

1. Magrath I, Adde M, Shad A, et al: Adults and children with small non-cleaved-cell lymphoma have a similar excellent out-come when treated with the same chemotherapy regimen. J Clin Oncol 14:925-934, 1996.
2. Mead GM, Sydes MR, Walewski J, et al: An international evaluation of CODOX-M and CODOX-M alternating with IVAC in adult Burkitt's lymphoma: Results of United Kingdom Lymphoma Group LY06 study. Ann Oncol 13:1264-1274, 2002.

PATIENT 3

A 35-year-old man with fever, jaundice, hepatosplenomegaly, and pancytopenia

A 35-year-old man with a past medical history significant for spontaneous splenic rupture 8 weeks prior, secondary to Epstein-Barr virus (EBV) infection, is admitted to the hospital. He is complaining of fatigue, anorexia, 20-lb weight loss, recurrent fevers, night sweats, and progressive jaundice.

Physical Examination: Temperature 38.8°C, pulse 96, blood pressure 106/50, pulse oximetry 90% on room air. HEENT: temporal wasting, icteric, mild pallor, submandibular adenopathy. Cardiovascular: regular rate and rhythm, without murmurs. Chest: dull percussion note with decreased breath sounds halfway up right lung. Abdomen: midline incision scar, inguinal adenopathy. Extremities: leg muscle wasting; no edema.

Laboratory Findings: Hemoglobin 8.2 g/dL, WBC 1700/μL, platelets 20,000/μL, reticulocytes 6%, haptoglobin less than 5%. Prothrombin time 15.9, INR 1.74, partial thromboplastin time 40. Ferritin greater than 2000. Biochemistry profile: electrolytes normal. BUN 10 mg/dL, creatinine 0.7 mg/dL, triglycerides 576. Liver function tests: ALT 50, AST 190, alkaline phosphatase 151 IU/L, total bilirubin 15.6 mg/dL, direct bilirubin 9.5 mg/dL, lactate dehydrogenase 921, albumin 2.3 g/dL. Chest radiograph: large right-sided pleural effusion. Bone marrow biopsy: numerous activated macrophages engulfing red blood cells, white blood cells, platelets, and precursor cells (see Figure).

Questions: What is the most likely diagnosis? What is the prognosis for this condition?

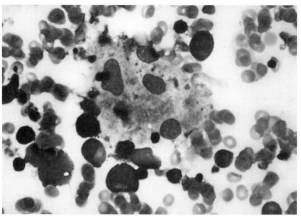

From Fisman DN: Hemophagocytic syndromes and infection. Emerg Infect Dis 6(6):601-608, 2000.

Answers: Epstein-Barr associated hemophagocytic lymphohistiocytosis (HLH) is the most likely diagnosis. The prognosis for this condition is poor.

Discussion: Hemophagocytic lymphohistiocytosis is a rare syndrome characterized by fever, splenomegaly, jaundice, and the pathological finding of phagocytosis by macrophages of erythrocytes, leukocytes, platelets, and their precursor cells. This phagocytosis is seen primarily in the bone marrow, spleen, liver, and lymph nodes. A familial form of HLH occurs in young children as an autosomal recessive disorder. In adults, a sporadic form of HLH occurs and has been associated with a variety of viral, bacterial, fungal, and parasitic infections. Connective tissue diseases and malignancies, particularly T-cell lymphomas, are also associated with sporadic HLH.

The clinical features of HLH include fever, splenomegaly, hepatomegaly, adenopathy, rash (typically maculopapular), and neurological signs. Seizures, meningismus, and encephalopathy are the commonly reported CNS features. Laboratory abnormalities include anemia, thrombocytopenia, neutropenia, and a biochemistry profile suggestive of hemolysis with hyperbilirubinemia and elevated lactate dehydrogenase. Most patients also have highly elevated serum ferritin and triglyceride levels. Serum fibrinogen levels are typically low, and there may be evidence of disseminated intravascular coagulation. The hallmark of the disease is the histopathological finding of hemophagocytosis in bone marrow, spleen, lymph nodes, and liver. Activated macrophages engulf erythrocytes, leukocytes, platelets, and their precursors.

A variety of infections are associated with HLH (see Table). Patients should have routine cultures of blood and urine as well as chest radiography. Serological testing for human immunodeficiency virus (HIV), Epstein-Barr virus, and cytomegalovirus (CMV) is also indicated. With the common association between T-cell lymphoma and HLH, T-cell receptor gene rearrangement studies should be performed on bone marrow to exclude an underlying lymphoma, even if an infection is confirmed.

Understanding the pathophysiology of EBV-associated HLH is instructive for optimal treatment strategy. Certain EBV subtypes infect and activate T-lymphocytes, inducing clonal expansion of these lymphocytes. Interferon-γ and tumor necrosis factor-α are produced in large amounts by the activated lymphocytes. These elaborated cytokines promote activation of macrophages and monocytes, with resulting phagocytosis of erythrocytes, neutrophils, platelets, and their precursors. Treatment strategies center on control of cytokine production, treatment of underlying infections, and eradication of the clonal population of EBV-infected lymphocytes by immunochemotherapy.

Because sporadic HLH is a rare condition, there are no controlled clinical trials to determine optimal therapy. Corticosteroids, cyclosporine, therapeutic apheresis, and intravenous immunoglobulin have been employed in an attempt to quell the "cytokine storm." Etoposide-based combination chemotherapy is used in an attempt to eradicate proliferating EBV-containing lymphocytes. Vigilance in eradicating any underlying infection is important; however, the addition of acyclovir has not been shown to be useful in the treatment of EBV-associated HLH. In non–EBV-associated HLH, supportive care and treatment of underlying infection lead to recovery in up to 65% of cases. EBV-associated HLH, however, has a dismal prognosis—it is almost always fatal.

In the present patient, T-cell receptor gene rearrangement studies suggested an underlying lymphoma. He was treated with a combination of steroids; intravenous immunoglobulin; plasmapheresis; broad-spectrum antibiotics; and cyclophosphamide, hydroxydaunomycin, Oncovin, and prednisone (CHOP) chemotherapy. Despite aggressive therapy, the patient continued to deteriorate. Progressive pancytopenia ensued, resulting in pulmonary hemorrhage and candida septicemia. He died of multiorgan failure 8 weeks after admission.

Infections Associated with Hemophagocytic Lymphohistiocytosis

Tuberculosis	Leishmaniasis
Histoplasmosis	Rickettsiosis
Malaria	Brucellosis
Salmonella typhi	Epstein-Barr virus
Cytomegalovirus	Parvovirus
Human immunodeficiency virus	Fungal infections

Clinical Pearls

1. Hemophagocytic lymphohistiocytosis (HLH) is a rare syndrome characterized by fever, splenomegaly, jaundice, and the pathological finding of phagocytosis by macrophages of erythrocytes, leukocytes, platelets, and their precursor cells.

2. The hallmark of the disease is the histopathological finding of hemophagocytosis in bone marrow, spleen, lymph nodes, and liver.

3. Sporadic HLH is associated with a number of infections, including EBV, HIV, and CMV.

REFERENCES

1. Fisman DN: Hemophagocytic syndromes and infection. Emerg Infect Dis 6(6):601-608, 2000.
2. Imashuku S: Advances in the management of hemophagocytic lymphohistiocytosis. Int J Hematol 72(1):1-11, 2000.

PATIENT 4

A 25-year-old man with respiratory distress and an anterior mediastinal mass

A 25-year-old previously healthy man in respiratory distress presents to the emergency department. He gives a 1-week history of progressive dyspnea, cough, and a feeling of fullness in his neck and face. During the month before admission, he had noticed malaise, night sweats, and significant weight loss.

Physical Examination: Temperature 37.5°C, pulse 110, blood pressure 140/90 mmHg. Respiration 32, pulse oximetry 85% on room air. General: tachypneic and distressed. HEENT: cyanotic, facial plethora. Neck: venous distention. Cardiovascular: regular rate and rhythm, without murmurs. Chest: stony dull percussion note and decreased fremitus with decreased breath sounds at both bases. Abdomen: no organomegaly, no ascites. Extremities: no edema or calf tenderness.

Laboratory Findings: Hemoglobin 12 g/dL, WBC 8000/μL, platelets 350,000/μL. Biochemistry profile: normal. Lactate dehydrogenase: 280. Chest CT scan: large anterior mediastinal mass with bilateral pleural effusions (see Figure). Biopsy of mediastinal mass: blastic-appearing cells that stain positively for terminal deoxynucleotidyl transferase (TdT).

Questions: What does the mediastinal mass most likely represent? What complication has occurred?

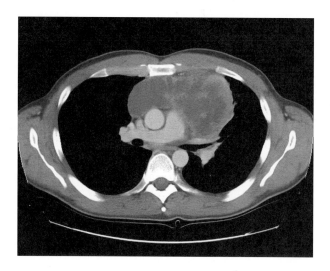

Diagnosis: The mediastinal mass represents lymphoblastic lymphoma complicated by the superior vena cava syndrome. The complication is acute respiratory distress due to superior vena-caval obstruction (SVCO).

Discussion: Lymphoblastic lymphoma represents 3 to 4% of all adult non-Hodgkin's lymphoma (NHL). It is much more common in children, in whom it represents 40% of NHL. Prognosis in adults is much poorer than in children. The peak incidence is in the second decade of life with a 2:1 male predominance.

Lymphoblastic lymphoma presents typically with symptomatic supradiaphragmatic adenopathy. A large anterior mediastinal mass is the classic presentation, and symptoms range from cough, wheezing, and dyspnea to respiratory distress. If the mediastinal mass is as large as 10 cm, SVCO syndrome, tracheal obstruction, and cardiac tamponade are frequent complications. Other malignancies that may present with a mediastinal mass include neuroendocrine tumors, Hodgkin's disease, germ cell tumors, sarcomas, thymoma, and other NHL, such as Burkitt's lymphoma and large-cell lymphoma.

Up to 90% of lymphoblastic lymphomas present with *stage III* or *IV* disease. Bone disease with bone pain, hypercalcemia, and lytic lesions may also be seen at presentation. Bone marrow involvement is seen in over 50% of cases. The incidence of central nervous system (CNS) disease at presentation is up to 20%, and there is a strong correlation between marrow involvement and CNS disease. The high rate of CNS disease at presentation necessitates spinal fluid evaluation and intrathecal methotrexate for CNS prophylaxis at the initial assessment.

Lymphoblastic lymphoma is sometimes difficult to distinguish from acute lymphocytic leukemia (ALL). In ALL, however, significant peripheral adenopathy is usually absent, and there is usually a high circulating blast count. Splenomegaly, which is usually absent in lymphoblastic lymphoma, is common and prominent in ALL. Peripheral blood and marrow involvement rarely produces thrombocytopenia in lymphoblastic lymphoma but is routinely seen in ALL. The finding of greater than 25% marrow lymphoblasts is, ultimately, diagnostic of leukemia.

Diagnostic studies required at presentation include: (a) a good history and physical, particularly noting the B-symptoms? unexplained and persistent symptoms of weight loss, night sweats, and fever; (b) a complete nodal assessment; (c) a routine blood profile with chemistry and LDH; (d) chest X-ray and CT imaging of chest, abdomen, and pelvis; (e) bone marrow aspirate and biopsy with TdT staining, immunophenotyping and karyotyping; (f) lumbar puncture with cytology;

(g) cytology of pleural fluid, if present; and (h) a bone scan and magnetic resonance imaging (MRI) of the CNS to assess for leptomeningeal disease.

The Ann Arbor Classification System is used for staging in adults. Cytological and lymph node biopsy demonstrate typically medium to large lymphoblasts with scant cytoplasm, moderately condensed nuclear chromatin, and an indistinct or small nucleoli. The lymphoblasts may be of T- or B-cell lineage. These two cell lines are morphologically indistinct but can be differentiated by immunophenotyping. Ninety percent of lymphoblastic lymphomas *stain positively for TdT*. TdT is a DNA polymerase that catalyzes the addition of random deoxynucleotides during Ig or T-cell receptor gene rearrangements. All other non-Hodgkin's lymphomas stain negatively for TdT.

Precursor B-cell lymphoblastic lymphoma expresses immunophenotypically B-cell markers, such as CD19, CD20, CD22, and CD34. Precursor T-cell lymphoblastic lymphoma is more common, and immunophenotyping is typically positive for CD3, CD5, and CD7. Immunophenotypically, lymphoblastic lymphoma is a very diverse disease; up to 30% of tumors express myeloid and lymphoid antigens. Immunophenotyping is thus generally not much use in prognostication. Karyotyping and chromosomal analysis have also not demonstrated reliable prognostic significance, except for the t(9;17) translocation, which has a more aggressive clinical course.

Typical features that are associated with a poor outcome in adults include: stage IV disease with either bone marrow or CNS disease, an elevated LDH (> 300), hyperleukocytosis, anemia at presentation (hemoglobin < 10), age greater than 30 years, B-symptoms, and any response less than a complete response to treatment.

The initial treatment of lymphoblastic lymphoma was modeled after standard NHL regimens, such as cyclophosphamid, hydroxydaunomycin, Oncovin, and prednisone (CHOP). Success with these regimens was limited, with typical complete response rates of 50% and disease-free survival limited to 25 to 50% of responders. With the success observed in pediatric populations using ALL regimes, a similar approach has been adopted in adults. *ALL-type regimes,* with their more intensive nature and longer maintenance phase, have resulted in an increase in the complete response rate of 75 to 90%, with long-term disease-free survival approaching 60% of initial responders. As the CNS is a frequent site of relapse, intensive intrathecal chemoprophylaxis is required. This is achieved typically using intrathecal methotrexate.

The role of allogenic and autologous bone marrow transplant has not been well established. In the many trials investigating the role of bone marrow transplant in lymphoblastic lymphoma, selection bias, application of different induction chemotherapy agents, and the heterogeneity of the disease limit firm conclusions. As the majority of patients achieve complete remission with conventional ALL treatment, bone marrow transplant should probably be reserved for patients who are in second remission, following relapse with conventional consolidation treatment.

The role of mediastinal irradiation is also not well established. Local radiation therapy carries the risk of cardiac toxicity, radiation pneumonitis, myelodysplasia, and secondary malignancies, such as breast cancer. Because the site of relapse is usually in the CNS or bone marrow, mediastinal radiation carries the risk of significant toxicity without clear benefit.

The present patient required intubation and mechanical ventilation for SVCO-induced acute respiratory distress. The SVCO responded to a combination of high-dose steroids and mediastinal irradiation, allowing prompt extubation. Cytological analysis of the pleural effusions demonstrated no evidence of lymphoma involvement. He is presently tolerating an ALL regimen, hyper CVAD (alternating cycles of cyclophosphamide, Adriamycin, vincristine, and steroids, rapidly followed by administration of methotrexate and high-dose cytosine arabinoside).

Clinical Pearls

1. Lymphoblastic lymphomas present typically with a large anterior mass.

2. Approximately 90% of patients with lymphoblastic lymphoma present with stage III or IV disease.

3. Ninety percent of lymphoblastic lymphomas stain positively for TdT.

4. Features associated with a poor outcome in adults include stage IV disease, an elevated LDH (> 300), hyperleukocytosis, anemia at presentation (hemoglobin < 10), age greater than 30, B-symptoms, and any response less than a complete response with initial treatment.

5. Prolonged courses of acute lymphocytic leukemia-like chemotherapy, with CNS prophylaxis using intrathecal methotrexate, has improved the disease-free and long-term survival of patients with lymphoblastic lymphoma.

REFERENCES

1. Thomas DA, Kantarjian HM: Lymphoblastic lymphoma. Hematol Oncol Clin North Am 15(1):51-95, 2001.
2. Hoelzer D, Gökbuget N, Digel W, et al: Outcome of adult patients with T-lymphoblastic lymphoma treated according to protocols for acute lymphoblastic leukemia. Blood 99:4379-4385, 2002.

PATIENT 5

A 75-year-old woman with persistent cough

A 75-year-old former smoker was well until a dry cough and progressive right-sided pleuritic chest pain developed 2 months ago. A chest X-ray demonstrates a right upper lobe infiltrate and a small right pleural effusion. These findings persist, despite an empirical course of antibiotics. A chest CT scan demonstrates a 3-cm stellate nodule within the right upper lobe, 2 subcentimeter nodules within the left lung, a moderate-sized right pleural effusion, and mediastinal lymphadenopathy. All of these findings are new compared to a screening chest CT scan obtained 3 years ago.

Physical Examination: General: thin; no acute distress. Temperature 36.1°C, pulse 90, blood pressure 110/50 mmHg. Cardiovascular: regular rate and rhythm without murmurs. Chest: clear to auscultation bilaterally. Abdomen: soft, nontender, no organomegaly, no masses. Back: no tenderness of vertebral spinous processes. Extremities: notable for clubbing of fingernails bilaterally.

Laboratory Findings: CBC, coagulation studies, and biochemistry profile: normal. Liver function tests: unremarkable. Diagnostic thoracentesis: pleural fluid positive for malignant cells consistent with squamous cell carcinoma.

Questions: What stage of lung cancer does this patient have? What treatment is recommended?

Answers: The patient has either stage IV or "wet IIIB" non–small-cell lung cancer. Combination chemotherapy is the recommended treatment, with the choice of regimen informed by comorbid conditions and patient preferences regarding potential toxicities.

Discussion: Non–small-cell lung cancer (NSCLC) is staged using the TNM system. Patients with NSCLC frequently develop pleural effusions that have no malignant cells on cytology. Given the poor diagnostic yield of cytology specimens obtained from thoracentesis, pleural effusions must be nonbloody, exudative, and have negative cytology on multiple cytopathological examinations to be excluded as a staging element in these patients. Consider video-assisted thoracoscopic surgery (VATS) and/or pleurodesis should be considered for symptomatic relief or prevention of recurrent effusions in these patients.

This patient has a cytopathologically positive pleural effusion, identifying the presence of stage IIIB disease, which is defined by either T_4 (primary tumor involving other named organs or great vessels within the chest, a satellite nodule within the primary tumor-bearing lobe of lung, or malignant pleural effusion) or N_3 disease (involvement of contralateral intrathoracic lymph nodes or involvement of any scalene or supraclavicular lymph nodes). The subset of these patients with malignant effusions are commonly said to have "wet IIIB" disease.

The presence of new contralateral nodules on this patient's chest CT makes the presence of stage IV disease likely. If this patient did not have a malignant pleural effusion, it would be prudent to biopsy a contralateral nodule to help define the presence of advanced disease. Because patients with wet IIIB disease have a similar prognosis and similar treatment options as patients with stage IV disease, and as a group are labeled as having "advanced" NSCLC, it is unnecessary to pursue further diagnostic studies to define this patient's stage.

Non–small-cell lung cancer has traditionally been viewed as a malignancy that affects primarily men. However, recent reports have demonstrated that this is not the case. Although lung cancer rates in men have been decreasing over the past 2 decades, the rate of lung cancer among women has steadily risen since the 1930s. Currently, lung cancer kills approximately 68,000 women annually, accounting for more deaths than those attributed to cancers of the breast, ovary, and uterus combined.

In patients with advanced NSCLC, the primary goals of therapy are prolongation of survival and palliation of symptoms to enhance the patient's quality of life. Meta-analyses have demonstrated that cisplatin-based doublets improve median survival, improve quality of life, and are cost-effective for patients with advanced NSCLC. Systemic chemotherapy is now considered a standard of care in the treatment of advanced NSCLC, as long as the patient is functionally independent and has no critical metastases that require site-specific interventions, such as palliative radiation therapy. The most commonly used chemotherapy doublets for advanced NSCLC include a platinum agent (cisplatin or carboplatin) added to either docetaxel, paclitaxel, gemcitabine, or vinorelbine. Numerous studies have demonstrated the superiority of platinum-based doublets to platinum monotherapy or to other chemotherapeutic agents given alone. Despite extensive evaluation, there is currently no standard role for the use of triplets of chemotherapy, which, despite improved response rates, lead to greater toxicity and no survival benefit. The role of radiotherapy for patients with advanced NSCLC is confined to palliation of symptoms, and there is currently no role for concurrent chemoradiotherapy in this setting.

Multiple recent phase III trials comparing these doublet regimens suggest similar efficacy in advanced NSCLC. In a large, randomized four-arm trial that compared cisplatin/docetaxel, cisplatin/gemcitabine, and carboplatin/paclitaxel versus a control arm of cisplatin plus 24-hour infusion paclitaxel, all three experimental doublets demonstrated efficacy outcomes similar to the reference regimen, with response rates ranging from 17 to 21%, median survivals of 8 months, and 1-year survival rates of 31 to 36%. Specific toxicities varied by treatment arm.

In the TAX 326 trial, the largest randomized trial in advanced NSCLC, three arms were compared: cisplatin/docetaxel and carboplatin/docetaxel versus a control arm of cisplatin/vinorelbine. Patients treated with cisplatin/docetaxel had a statistically significant higher response rate (31.6% vs 24.5%) and median survival (11.3 months vs 10.1 months) compared with the control arm. Although the carboplatin/docetaxel arm demonstrated nonstatistically significant inferior results compared to the control arm, the trial was not structured to make a direct comparison of cisplatin/docetaxel versus carboplatin/docetaxel. Toxicity was similar in all three arms. This trial is appropriately cited as support for the superiority of cisplatin/docetaxel over cisplatin/vinorelbine in advanced NSCLC. It has also been interpreted by some oncologists as evidence of cisplatin's superiority over carboplatin when combined with docetaxel, although this remains controversial.

Active areas of investigation include the role of nonplatinum-containing doublets as primary therapy and appropriate treatment of the elderly. In clinical practice, the choice of which doublet to use remains a decision that should be made on an individualized basis, informed by nonefficacy issues, such as cost, convenience, and toxicity.

More recently, novel targeted therapies directed at the epidermal growth factor receptor (EGFR), such as gefitinib (Iressa) and erlotinib (Tarceva), have been developed. These oral agents inhibit phosphorylation of the tyrosine kinase located within the intracytoplasmic tail of the EGFR and thereby reduce downstream messages that stimulate cellular growth, proliferation, and invasion. Used as a single agent administered on a daily schedule, gefitinib offers a 10 to 15% response rate and 40% rate of symptomatic improvement regardless of patients' performance status or number of prior therapies. Responses are generally evident within 1 month. In contrast to chemotherapy, treatment with these agents is associated with limited toxicity, largely confined to acneiform rash and diarrhea. Three groups of patients most likely to respond to these agents are women, never-smokers (less than 100 lifetime cigarettes), and those with histology consistent with bronchoalveolar carcinoma. Recent reports suggest that the presence of activating mutations within the tyrosine kinase domain of the EGFR may best predict responsiveness to these agents.

Clinical Pearls

1. "Wet" stage IIIB and stage IV non–small-cell lung cancer (NSCLC) have similar prognoses and treatment options and are appropriately grouped together as "advanced" NSCLC.

2. Combination chemotherapy remains the foundation of treatment for patients with advanced NSCLC. Decisions about what specific doublet to use are often informed by nonefficacy issues, such as potential toxicity and convenience.

3. Clinical predictors of response to tyrosine kinase inhibitors of the epidermal growth factor receptor (EGFR) include female gender, never-smoker history, and bronchoalveolar carcinoma histology. Activating mutations within the EGFR–tyrosine kinase domain appear to be powerful molecular predictors of response.

REFERENCES

1. Mountain CF: Revisions in the international system for staging lung cancer. Chest 111(6):1710-1717, 1997.
2. Schiller JH, Harrington D, Belani CP, et al: for the Eastern Cooperative Oncology Group. Comparison of four chemotherapy regimens for advanced non-small cell lung cancer. N Engl J Med 346(2):92-98, 2002.
3. Fossella F, Pereira JR, von Pawel J, et al: Randomized, multinational, phase III study of docetaxel plus platinum combinations versus vinorelbine plus cisplatin for advanced non-small-cell lung cancer: The TAX 326 Study Group. J Clin Oncol 21(16):3016-3024, 2003.
4. Kris MG, Natale RB, Herbst RS, et al: Efficacy of gefitinib, an inhibitor of the epidermal growth factor receptor tyrosine kinase, in symptomatic patients with non-small cell lung cancer: A randomized trial. JAMA 290(16):2149-2158, 2003.
5. Lynch TJ, Bell DW, Sordella R, et al: Activating mutations in the epidermal growth factor receptor underlying responsiveness of non-small cell lung cancer to gefitinib. N Engl J Med 350(21):2129-2139, 2004.
6. Patel JD, Bach PB, Kris M: Lung cancer in U.S. women: A contemporary epidemic. JAMA 291(14):1763-1768, 2004.

PATIENT 6

A 77-year-old man with lymphocytosis, anemia, and thrombocytopenia

A 77-year-old man with a past medical history significant for coronary artery disease has had a positive stress test and presents with lymphocytosis, anemia, and thrombocytopenia on a routine CBC prior to an angiogram.

Physical Examination: Temperature 36.4°C, pulse 56, blood pressure 142/58 mmHg. General: obese. HEENT: anicteric, no tonsillar enlargement. Cardiovascular: mild bradycardia, regular rhythm, 2/6 systolic ejection murmur at apex. Chest: clear to auscultation. Abdomen: soft, no hepato-splenomegaly. Extremities: trace ankle edema, no ulcerations. Lymph nodes: 1.5 cm left and 0.8 cm right axillary lymphadenopathy.

Laboratory Findings: Hemoglobin 11.4 g/dL, WBC 47,900/μL, platelets 142,000/μL, lympho-cytes 86%, reticulocytes 0.8%. Peripheral blood smear: increased number of mature lymphocytes (see Figure). Peripheral flow cytometry: monoclonal B-cell lymphoid population representing about 84% of total blood cells, staining with moderate intensity for CD20 λ-light chain, positive for CD5, DC19, CD23, and CD52; and negative for CD10, CD38, and CD103.

Questions: What is the most likely diagnosis? What is the next step in management?

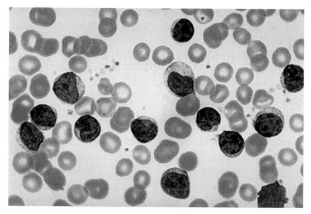

Printed with permission of Edward C. Klatt, MD, Webpath, University of Utah.

Answers: Chronic lymphocytic leukemia, Rai stage I, is the most likely diagnosis. The appropriate management is observation.

Discussion: Chronic lymphocytic leukemia (CLL) represents 25% of all leukemias and is thus the most common kind. In 2003, approximately 7300 people were diagnosed with CLL, and 4400 died of the disease. Median age at diagnosis has decreased to 62, likely due to detection of asymptomatic cases on routine CBC. Survival is approximately 73% at 5 years. The risk factors are not clear, but some studies note familial incidence of leukemias or lymphomas in up to 20% of CLL patients.

At the time of diagnosis 20 to 25% of patients are asymptomatic—especially if diagnosed incidentally, as was the patient in this case. B-symptoms, consisting of fever greater than 38°C, drenching night sweats, or weight loss greater than 10% are seen in only 5 to 10% at presentation. Most patients have lymphadenopathy, over half have splenomegaly, some have hepatomegaly. Laboratory data show lymphocytosis of at least 5000/μL, over 100,000 cells in 30% of the patients. The lymphocytes appear to be of normal size and maturity. Other abnormalities may include mild anemia and thrombocytopenia, positive Coombs' test, and hypogammaglobulinemia.

Although the CLL cells may appear morphologically mature, they are, in fact, developmentally delayed and immunologically incompetent. They produce autoantibodies responsible for autoimmune hemolytic anemia in 11% of CLL patients and autoimmune thrombocytopenia in 2 to 3%. There is also increased risk of other hematological and solid malignancies that require attention to routine preventive care. Because CLL cells do not produce functional immunoglobulins, patients are at risk for upper respiratory infections and, later in the course, for herpes zoster.

At least 95% of the time, the malignant CLL clone originates from a B-cell, as reflected in the typical B-cell markers found on the surface by immunohistochemical staining or by flow cytometry: CD19, CD20 (weakly expressed), CD21, CD23, and CD24. An extremely low level of surface membrane immunoglobulin with a single light chain expression confirms clonality. CLL cells also express a T-cell marker, CD5. There are no pathognomonic cytogenetic abnormalities, but trisomy 12 and deletions in 17p, 11q, and 13q can be seen and are of prognostic significance. Poor prognostic factors include diffuse pattern of bone marrow infiltration, lymphocyte doubling time of less than 1 year, deletion 17p (associated with p53 mutation), deletion 118, expression of CD38 and presence of unmutated rearranged immunoglobin heavy chain variable-region (vr) gene (signifying origin from a pregerminal center B-cell), and expression of ZAP-70.

Rai and Modified Rai Staging for Chronic Lymphocytic Leukemia

Stage: Rai; Modified Rai (Survival)	Definition
0; Low (> 10 yr)*	Lymphocytosis (peripheral or bone marrow)
1; Intermediate (6 yr)	L + lymphadenopathy
2; Intermediate (6 yr)	L + hepatomegaly or splenomegaly
3; High (2 yr)	L + anemia (hemoglobin < 11)
4; High (2 yr)	L + thrombocytopenia (platelets < 100)

*50% of presenting patients.
L = lymphocytosis.

The best known staging system in CLL is Rai, now often modified for simplicity and similarity in survival impact (see Table). Binet staging corresponds roughly to modified Rai. The present patient has stage I CLL, consisting of lymphocytosis and lymphadenopathy. At this stage, observation is appropriate.

The need for treatment is dictated chiefly by anemia and thrombocytopenia, after autoimmune causes have been ruled out. Extreme symptoms, such as symptomatic lymphadenopathy and autoimmune hemolytic anemia or immune thrombocytopenia refractory to treatment, are also indications for treatment. Fludarabine is the main treatment agent, with other purine analogs, such as cladribine and pentostatin in trials. Rituximab is often added, even though CLL cells have weak CD20 expression. Oral chlorambucil is the old agent of choice, which should still be used, if the patient is physiologically older and has decreased performance status.

Clinical Pearls

1. Chronic lymphocytic leukemia (CLL) is a common leukemia of B-cell–like origin. Diagnosis requires persistent peripheral lymphocytosis of over 5000/μL.

2. CLL diagnosis is usually confirmed on peripheral flow cytometry. Cells are positive for CD5 and for at least one B-cell marker, such as CD19, CD20, CD21, CD23, or CD24, and have weak expression of surface membrane immunoglobulin with light chain restriction. Bone marrow is usually not necessary.

3. CLL cells are immunologically incompetent. The patient is at risk for upper respiratory infections and herpes zoster; autoimmune hemolytic anemia and thrombocytopenia; and increased risk of other malignancies.

4. CLL is more heterogeneous than previously thought. Prognosis is increasingly guided by phenotypic description and cytogenetic abnormalities.

5. Main indications for treatment are anemia and thrombocytopenia. Treatment is with fludarabine or chlorambucil, sometimes with the addition of rituximab.

REFERENCES

1. Dohner H, Stilgenbauer S, Benner A, et al: Genomic aberrations and survival in chronic lymphocytic leukemia. N Engl J Med 343(26):1910-1916, 2000.
2. Rai KR, Peterson BL, Appelbaum FR, et al: Fludarabine compared with chlorambucil as primary therapy for chronic lymphocytic leukemia. N Engl J Med 343:1750-1757, 2000.
3. Keating MJ, Chiorazzi N, Messmer B, et al: Biology and treatment of chronic lymphocytic leukemia. American Society of Hematology Education book: Hematology. Washington, DC, ASH, 2003, pp 153-175.

PATIENT 7

A 44-year-old man with pancytopenia and splenomegaly

A 42-year-old man reports an increased incidence of nontraumatic bruising and exercise intolerance. He also notes a new onset of cough associated with mild hemoptysis. He presents to his internist who performs a CBC that reveals pancytopenia. The patient denies any recent history of fever.

Physical Examination: General: well-appearing. HEENT: petechial hemorrhage on tip of tongue. Lymph nodes: no palpable adenopathy. Cardiac: regular rate and rhythm. Chest: clear to auscultation. Abdomen: soft, nontender, with spleen tip palpated 3 cm below left costal margin; no hepatomegaly noted. Extremities: no clubbing, cyanosis, or edema. Skin: petechial hemorrhages on right hand and pretibial areas bilaterally.

Laboratory Findings: Hemoglobin 11 g/dL, platelets 60,000/μL, WBC 18,500/μL, absolute neutrophils 0.3/μL. Peripheral blood smear: predominance of atypical lymphoid cells with abundant cytoplasm and evidence of cytoplasmic projections (see Figure). Bone marrow aspirate and biopsy: lymphocytic infiltrate positive for CD20 and CD25. Abdominal ultrasound: mild splenomegaly.

Questions: What is the most likely cause of this patient's pancytopenia? What is the treatment for this condition?

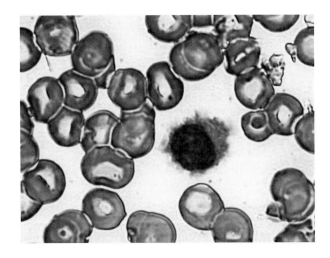

Answers: Hairy cell leukemia is most likely the cause. Chlorodeoxyadenosine (CdA) is the treatment of choice.

Discussion: Hairy cell leukemia (HCL) is an unusual B-cell malignancy characterized by pancytopenia, splenomegaly, and the presence of cells in the peripheral blood, spleen, and bone marrow with hair-like cytoplasmic projections. It represents about 2% of all leukemias. The mean age of presentation is 50 years, with a male:female ratio of approximately 4:1.

At presentation, weakness, weight loss, and dyspnea are the most common symptoms. Increased bruising secondary to thrombocytopenia and bacterial infections due to granulocytopenia are also frequently seen. Palpable splenomegaly is present in 85% of patients. Although uncommon at presentation, significant abdominal lymphadenopathy may be seen in up to 15% of patients during the course of their illness.

About two-thirds of patients have pancytopenia at diagnosis. Most patients have leucopenia, but occasional patients have a normal WBC count. Rarely, patients have an extreme leukocytosis of greater than 200,000/μL; this extreme elevation is seen typically in the variant form of hairy cell leukemia. Most patients have neutropenia and monocytopenia.

The disease is diagnosed by its typical peripheral blood morphology with *cytoplasmic projections* on the cell surface. Hairy cells contain large amounts of tartrate-resistant acid phosphatase (TRAP). Therefore, TRAP cytochemistry is an important diagnostic investigation. Immunophenotyping demonstrates the presence in the blood or bone marrow of a clonal population of mature B-cells expressing CD19, CD20, CD22, FMC7 with the hairy cell markers CD11c, CD25, and CD103. The cells lack typically CD5, CD10, and CD23, allowing differentiation from chronic lymphocytic leukemia and follicular lymphoma.

The bone marrow is inaspirable in 50% of cases. The marrow biopsy has typically a focal or diffuse infiltrate of leukemic cells. Characteristically, the hairy cell nuclei are surrounded by a clear zone of cytoplasm, giving the so-called "halo" appearance. Another unusual feature of the HCL marrow is the presence of *reticulin fibrosis*.

Two diseases that may be mistaken for HCL are splenic lymphoma with villous lymphocytes (SLVL) and the hairy cell leukemia variant (HCL-V). Patients with HCL-V present at an average age of 70. They have typically a high leucocyte count and do not have neutropenia or monocytopenia. Also, in contrast to the cells in HCL, the variant hairy cells are characteristically CD25 negative. Patients with SLVL have circulating malignant cells that closely resemble hairy cells. These patients also typically have massive splenomegaly. Marrow function is often well preserved, and monocytopenia is not a feature. In contrast to the cells in HCL, the SLVL cells are negative for CD103.

In asymptomatic patients, treatment should be delayed. Common indications for treatment include symptomatic splenomegaly, cytopenia, and the leukemic phase of hairy cell leukemia (WBC greater than 20,000/μL). Purine analogs, such as chlorodeoxyadenosine (CdA) and deoxycoformycin (dCF), are the treatment of choice. Cladribine (CdA) is highly effective in the treatment of HCL. Almost all patients respond to a single course, administered over 7 consecutive days at a dose of 0.09 mg/kg per day by continuous infusion. The major toxicity of CdA is marrow suppression and a high incidence of neutropenic fever. Pentostatin (dCF) is usually given at 4 mg/m^2 by intravenous infusion every other week. Neutropenia and fever are also seen with pentostatin. Both nucleoside analogs can cause a prolonged depletion of CD4+ T-cells. Prophylaxis against *Pneumocystis carinii* pneumonia with cotrimoxazole is often practiced. In disease that is refractory to purine analog treatment, a recombinant immunotoxin targeted against the CD22 antigen of hairy cells can induce a complete remission.

The present patient was treated with a single course of cladribine. The course was complicated by an episode of febrile neutropenia requiring admission and antibiotics. He continues to be in a complete hematological remission 2 years after treatment.

Clinical Pearls

1. Hairy cell leukemia (HCL) is an unusual B-cell malignancy characterized by pancytopenia, splenomegaly, and the presence of cells in the peripheral blood, spleen, and bone marrow with hair-like cytoplasmic projections.

2. Immunophenotyping demonstrates the presence in the blood or bone marrow of a clonal population of mature B-cells expressing CD19, CD20, CD22, and FMC7 with the hairy cell markers CD11c, CD25, and CD103.

3. The bone marrow is inaspirable in 50% of cases.

4. Purine analogs, such as chlorodeoxyadenosine (CdA) and deoxycoformycin (dCF), are the treatment of choice for HCL.

REFERENCES

1. Allsup DJ, Cawley JC: The diagnosis and treatment of hairy-cell leukemia. Blood Rev 16:225-262, 2002.
2. Andrey J, Savan A: Therapeutic advances in the treatment of hairy cell leukemia. Leuk Res 25:361-368, 2000.
3. Kreitman RJ, Wilson HW, Bergeron K, et al: Efficacy of the anti-CD22 recombinant immunotoxin BL22 in chemotherapy-resistant hairy-cell leukemia. N Engl J Med 345(4):241-247, 2001.

PATIENT 8

A 53-year-old man with fever, night sweats, and weight loss

A 53-year-old man presents with a 3-month history of fever, night sweats, and 40-pound weight loss. A month prior to his initial evaluation he had noticed left-sided substernal chest pain and dyspnea on exertion. A prior cardiac evaluation for chest pain revealed no evidence of coronary artery disease. The patient has a long history of tobacco use.

Physical Examination: General: well-appearing. Temperature 37.5°C. HEENT: anicteric, mucous membranes moist. Lymph nodes: no palpable adenopathy. Cardiac: regular rate and rhythm. Pulmonary: clear to auscultation bilaterally. Abdomen: soft, nontender. Extremities: no edema or cyanosis.

Laboratory Findings: CBC: normal. Chemistry panel: normal. CT scan of chest: multiple pulmonary nodules and a dominant left pleural-based mass (see Figure). Video-assisted thoracoscopic surgical biopsy: positive for cellular infiltrate composed of histiocytic cells staining positively for CD1a and S100.

Question: What is this patient's diagnosis?

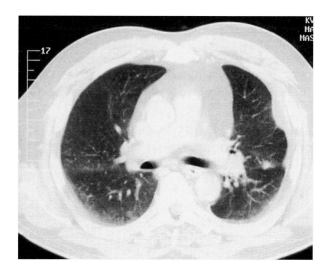

Diagnosis: Pulmonary Langerhans-cell histiocytosis is the diagnosis.

Discussion: Pulmonary Langerhans-cell histiocytosis (PLCH) is a rare disorder that is part of a spectrum of diseases characterized by monoclonal proliferation and infiltration of organs by Langerhans cells. Langerhans-cell histiocytoses (LCH) are classified as LCH with single-organ involvement (PLCH) or LCH with multiorgan or multisystem disease. Localized forms of LCH were previously referred to as eosinophilic granuloma, whereas multisystem diseases were referred to by a variety of names, such as systemic histiocytosis X, Letterer-Siwe disease, and Hand-Schüller-Christian disease.

The most consistent epidemiological association with PLCH is cigarette smoking, with up to 90% of patients giving a history of tobacco use. At present there are no known genetic risk factors that predispose to PLCH.

Normal Langerhans cells (LC) are differentiated antigen-presenting cells of monocyte-macrophage lineage. In LCH, clonal expansion has been demonstrated using probes that identify patterns of X-chromosome inactivation. On histology, LC in LCH are rounded instead of the usual dendritic shape. They also display increased numbers of Birbeck granules, which appear as pentalaminar (five-layered), rod-shaped intracellular structures when visualized by electron microscopy. Immunohistochemical studies are useful in recognizing LC, which stain for the S100 protein, CD1a, and HLA-DR.

Patients with PLCH present in a variety of ways. The most common presentation is with a nonproductive cough and dyspnea. Pleuritic chest pain is an infrequent finding. Constitutional symptoms, such as weight loss, fever, night sweats, and anorexia, occur in up to a third of patients. Involvement of other organs occurs in up to 15% of patients and can result in bone pain. Polyuria and polydipsia with diabetes insipidus is related to hypothalamic or posterior pituitary involvement. The physical examination is usually unremarkable, although with disease progression, clubbing and cor pulmonale may be observed.

Pulmonary function testing in patients with PLCH demonstrates usually mild obstructive, restrictive, or mixed abnormalities. A decreased carbon monoxide lung diffusion (DLCO) is present in 60 to 90% of patients. The chest radiograph is abnormal in most patients, demonstrating typically micronodular or reticulonodular and interstitial infiltrates, predominantly affecting middle and upper lung lobes. As the disease progresses, the number of radiographic nodules decreases, and cystic changes become more prominent. The cystic and nodular changes are better visualized with high-resolution CT. The combination of diffuse, irregularly shaped cystic spaces with small peri-bronchiolar nodular opacities, predominantly affecting the middle and upper lobes in a patient with an extensive smoking history, is highly suggestive of PLCH. Late-stage disease is characterized by honeycombing in the upper lungs.

Bronchoalveolar lavage (BAL) demonstrates typically increased numbers of Langerhans cells in the BAL fluid. These cells are identified by positive staining with antibodies against CD1a. The diagnosis of PLCH is very likely, if greater than 5% of BAL fluid cells stain positively for CD1a. Because transbronchoscopic lung biopsy has a low diagnostic yield, video-assisted thoracoscopic biopsy is often required to confirm the tissue diagnosis.

Smoking cessation is an essential part of the management of this disease. Occasional patients have objective radiographic and physiological improvement in lung function after smoking cessation. Bronchogenic cancers and progression of chronic obstructive lung disease are seen more commonly in patients who continue to smoke heavily.

Corticosteroids are the mainstay of medical management of PLCH. Several anecdotal reports and case series suggest that corticosteroid therapy results in the stabilization of the disease with symptomatic improvement. However, there are no well-designed randomized trials confirming a benefit of steroid therapy to smoking cessation alone. Chemotherapy agents, such as vinblastine, methotrexate, cyclophosphamide, etoposide, and cladribine, have been used in patients with progressive disease that is unresponsive to corticosteroids.

In a review by Vassallo and colleagues of over 100 patients with PLCH, the overall median survival was 12.5 years, which was significantly shorter than matched patients of the same sex and age. Variables predictive of a shorter survival included older age, a lower FEV_1, a higher residual volume, a lower ratio of FEV_1 to forced vital capacity, and a reduced carbon monoxide diffusing capacity. Progressive respiratory failure was the cause of death in 15 of the 33 deaths in this patient cohort.

The present patient was initially treated with a course of corticosteroids, but radiological and symptomatic response was minimal. He was subsequently treated with vinblastine and concurrent steroids followed by single agent 6-mercaptopurine. The response was excellent. He is presently continuing treatment with oral methotrexate.

Clinical Pearls

1. Pulmonary Langerhans-cell histiocytosis (PLCH) is a rare disorder that is part of a spectrum of diseases characterized by monoclonal proliferation and infiltration of organs by Langerhans cells (LC).

2. The most consistent epidemiological association with PLCH is cigarette smoking.

3. Immunohistochemical studies are useful in recognizing LC, which stain for the S100 protein, CD1a, and HLA-DR.

4. A decreased DLCO on pulmonary function testing is present in 60 to 90% of patients with PLCH.

5. Smoking cessation and corticosteroids are the mainstay of management of PLCH.

REFERENCES

1. Vasallo R, Ryu JH, Colby TV, et al: Pulmonary Langerhans cell histiocytosis. N Engl J Med 342:1969-1978, 2000.
2. Vasallo R, Ryu JH, Schroeder DR, et al: Clinical outcome of pulmonary Langerhans-cell histiocytosis in adults. N Engl J Med 346:484-490, 2002.
3. Sundar KM, Gosselin MV, Chung HL, et al: Pulmonary Langerhans cell histiocytosis: Emerging concepts in pathobiology, radiology, and clinical evolution of disease. Chest 123:1673-1683, 2003.

PATIENT 9

A 27-year-old man with fatigue, left upper quadrant discomfort, and eosinophilia

A 27-year-old man presents to his physician complaining of mild fatigue and left upper quadrant discomfort. He also complains of some facial flushing on occasion but denies night sweats or weight loss. He gives no history of recent foreign travel and has an otherwise negative past medical history.

Physical Examination: General: well-appearing. HEENT: slight facial flushing. Temperature 36.6°C. Lymph nodes: no adenopathy. Cardiac: regular rate and rhythm, no murmurs or gallop. Chest: clear to auscultation. Abdomen: 2-cm spleen tip palpated at costal margin. Extremities: no clubbing, cyanosis, or edema. Skin: blanching erythematous rash over face, trunk, and arms.

Laboratory Findings: WBC 30,100/μL, hemoglobin 14.4 g/dL, platelets 341,000/μL; differential count significant for 39.8% eosinophils. Chemistry profile: normal. HIV testing: negative. RPR: negative. Hepatitis serology: negative. Peripheral blood smear: normal red cell morphology with marked eosinophilia. Bone marrow biopsy: hypercellular marrow with marked increased myeloid and megakaryocytopoiesis. Myeloid cells are seen in all maturation stages with significant eosinophilia. Cytogenetics: normal. FISH (fluorescent *in situ* hybridization): no evidence of BCR-ABL.

Question: What is the most likely diagnosis?

Diagnosis: Idiopathic hypereosinophilic syndrome is the likely diagnosis.

Discussion: The hypereosinophilic syndromes are a rare group of hematological disorders characterized by sustained overproduction of eosinophils in the bone marrow, eosinophilia, tissue infiltration, and organ damage. A patient presenting with peripheral blood eosinophilia should be evaluated for an underlying condition, such as parasitic infection, allergic reaction, malignancy, and rheumatologic disorders. When these conditions are excluded, the diagnosis of idiopathic hypereosinophilic syndrome (HES) should be considered.

The diagnostic criteria for HES includes: sustained eosinophilia (more than 1500 eosinophils per cubic millimeter for more than 6 months; the absence of other causes of eosinophilia; and signs of organ involvement, including the heart, central and peripheral nervous system, lungs, and skin. The release of eosinophilic granule contents may lead to direct endothelial damage, causing fibrosis or thrombosis. Cardiac involvement can result in mural thrombosis or Loeffler's endomyocarditis (a condition characterized by endomyocardial thickening due to fibrosis leading to ventricular cavity compromise). Dermatologic symptoms include rash, urticaria, and angioedema. Hepatosplenomegaly diarrhea and colitis are also seen. Fatigue, myalgia, and fever are frequently described.

The syndrome is more common in men (9:1) and occurs in the 3rd to 5th decades of life. There are at least two distinct subsets of patients with HES: Those with a myeloproliferative-like disease and those with a clonal population of lymphocytes overproducing eosinophilic cytokines. Patients with the myeloproliferative presentation may develop chronic eosinophilic leukemia or transform to acute myeloid leukemia. The lymphocytic variant of HES is caused by a monoclonal expansion of T-lymphocytes, resulting in excess secretion of IL-5. The lymphocytic variant of HES is commonly associated with cutaneous involvement. Numerous cytogenetic abnormalities have been described in HES; however, most patients are found to have a normal karyotype.

Although the disease is often chronic and indolent, it is more frequently progressive and, in some instances, may be rapidly fatal. Organ damage is usually steadily progressive, with congestive heart failure resulting from endomyocardial fibrosis involving the valve leaflets. Treatment of HES attempts to limit organ damage by controlling the eosinophil count. Traditionally, steroids have been the initial treatment of choice. Steroid-unresponsive patients are often treated with cytotoxic therapy, such as hydroxyurea, vincristine, and cyclophosphamide. Interferon-α is also effective in eliciting durable hematologic and cytogenetic responses in HES.

It has been reported that some patients with HES respond to Imatinib mesylate (Gleevec). This tyrosine kinase inhibitor has revolutionized therapy for chronic myeloid leukemia (CML), with over 90% of previously untreated patients in the chronic phase achieving a complete hematologic response and 70% achieving a complete cytogenetic response after 1 year of therapy. Imatinib not only inhibits the ABL tyrosine kinase inhibitor in CML but also has been found to inhibit other tyrosine kinase inhibitors, such as KIT and PDGFRA. Imatinib is also active in the treatment of gastrointestinal stromal tumors, which frequently harbor activating mutations in the KIT gene. Coley and colleagues reported that 9 of 11 HES patients treated with Imatinib achieved a complete hematologic response lasting more than 3 months. Further molecular characterization of these patients revealed no evidence of activating mutations in KIT, PDGFRA, or PDGFRB. However, these researchers identified a deletion breakpoint on the long arm of chromosome 4 not evident on standard karyotyping, resulting in the kinase domain of PDGFRA fusing to a gene named FIP1L1. The fusion protein FIP1L1-PDGFRA is a constitutively active tyrosine kinase that is inhibited by Imatinib. This fusion gene was subsequently detected in 9 of 16 patients with HES and in 5 of 9 patients with responses to Imatinib.

The present patient was treated with Imatinib, with some improvement in his symptoms of facial flushing and fatigue. His eosinophil count, however, remained elevated.

Clinical Pearls

1. A patient presenting with peripheral blood eosinophilia should be evaluated for an underlying condition, such as parasitic infection, allergic reaction, malignancy, and rheumatologic conditions. When these conditions are excluded, the diagnosis of idiopathic hypereosinophilic syndrome (HES) should be considered.

2. The release of eosinophilic granule contents may lead to direct endothelial damage, causing fibrosis, including Loeffler's endomyocarditis.

3. The fusion protein FIP1L1-PDGFRA is a constitutively active tyrosine kinase that is responsible for a proportion of HES cases.

4. Imatinib mesylate may result in a durable, complete hematologic response in patients with HES.

REFERENCES

1. Cools J, DeAngelo DJ, Gotlib J, et al: A tyrosine kinase created fusion of the PDGFRA and FIP1L1 genes as a therapeutic target of imatinib in idiopathic hypereosinophilic syndrome. N Engl J Med 348:1201-1214, 2003.
2. Coutre S, Gotlib J: Targeted treatment of hypereosinophilic syndromes and chronic eosinophilic leukemias with imatinib mesylate. Semin Cancer Biol 14(1):23-31, 2004.

PATIENT 10

A 63-year-old man with an elevated erythroid sedimentation rate and an immunoglobulin M (IgM) monoclonal gammopathy

A 63-year-old man with a past medical history significant for emphysema, diabetes mellitus, osteoporosis, and a remote history of colon cancer requiring adjuvant 5-FU/leucovorin chemotherapy was noted to have an elevated ESR on routine lab tests performed by his primary care physician.

Physical Examination: General: well-appearing. Vital signs: stable. HEENT: anicteric, no thyroid swelling. Lymph nodes: no palpable adenopathy. Cardiac: regular rate and rhythm. Abdomen: no tenderness or hepatosplenomegaly. Extremities: no clubbing, cyanosis, or edema.

Laboratory Findings: Hemoglobin 14.4 g/dL, WBC 6300/μL, platelets 196/μL. Chemistry panel: within normal limits. Total serum protein: normal. Serum protein electrophoresis: IgM monoclonal gammopathy of 3480 mg/dL. CT scan chest and abdomen: no evidence of adenopathy or splenomegaly. Bone marrow aspirate and biopsy: intratrabecular monoclonal lymphoplasmacytic infiltrate. Immunophenotyping is positive for CD19, CD20, CD22, cytoplasmic immunoglobulin, and FMC7. Stains for CD5, CD10, and CD23 are negative.

Questions: What is the most likely diagnosis? What additional tests will be useful to determine the prognosis for this man's condition?

Answers: Lymphoplasmacytoid lymphoma (Waldenström's macroglobulinemia) is the most likely diagnosis. A high β_2-microglobulin level and low serum albumin are associated with a worse prognosis.

Discussion: Waldenström's macroglobulinemia (WM) is a low-grade neoplasm of lymphocytic and plasmacytic cells that secrete a monoclonal immunoglobulin M (IgM). The disease occurs at a median age of 63 and is more common in men. Infiltration of the bone marrow by the neoplastic clone leads to cytopenia. Infiltration of other organs, including lymph nodes, liver, and spleen, results in lymphadenopathy and hepatosplenomegaly. Rarely, the dermis is infiltrated by malignant lymphoplasmacytic cells, resulting in nodular and macular lesions. This association of an IgM monoclonal protein with erythematous, urticarial skin lesions is known as Schnitzler's syndrome. Unlike multiple myeloma, lytic bone lesions are typically absent.

Circulating IgM monoclonal proteins can result in symptoms associated with hyperviscosity and cryoglobulinemia. Hyperviscosity occurs in 15% of patients and is clinically characterized by epistaxis, retinal hemorrhage, and headache. A diagnosis of symptomatic hyperviscosity should be treated with plasmapheresis. Approximately 25% of patients with WM have neurological abnormalities, including peripheral neuropathy, encephalopathy, and subarachnoid hemorrhage.

By definition the serum IgM is elevated in macroglobulinemia; the IgG is reduced in 60% of patients, and the IgA is reduced in about 20% of patients. Immunofixation is recommended to further characterize the type of light and heavy chains present. The light chain of the monoclonal IgM is κ in 75% of patients. Increased plasma volume is a frequent finding and results in low hemoglobin and hematocrit values. Transfusing blood in this setting can exacerbate symptoms of hyperviscosity. A spuriously high ESR is another frequent hematologic manifestation of WM.

The marrow aspirate is often hypocellular; however, the biopsy is typically hypercellular and diffusely infiltrated with lymphocytes, plasmacytoid lymphocytes, and plasma cells. The typical immunophenotype of WM consists of expression of pan-B-cell surface markers (CD19, CD20, CD22), cytoplasmic immunoglobulin, FMC7, CD38, and CD79a. WM can be differentiated from B-cell lymphocytic leukemia by the absence of the characteristic CLL markers, CD5, and CD23. A CT scan of the abdomen and pelvis to detect organomegaly and adenopathy is indicated. In the absence of symptoms, skeletal surveys and bone scans are not indicated.

The most common differential diagnosis of an IgM monoclonal protein is an IgM monoclonal gammopathy of undetermined significance (MGUS). It is not always straightforward to distinguish patients with this diagnosis. Patients with IgM-MGUS usually have no symptoms or signs, an IgM protein of less than 30 g/L, and a normal serum viscosity. Definitive distinction between the two diseases is often concluded by the need for treatment in WM. An elevated serum IgM can also be detected in patients with a variety of other lymphoid neoplasms, including malignant lymphoma and multiple myeloma. The differentiation between IgM multiple myeloma and WM is predominantly based on the lytic lesions, hypercalcemia, and the more frequent finding of renal insufficiency seen in multiple myeloma.

WM is an incurable disease. Therapy should thus be focused on palliation of symptoms. Observation of asymptomatic patients is preferred. Treatment is indicated for patients with anemia, symptoms of hyperviscosity, lymphadenopathy, hepatosplenomegaly, bleeding, or neurological symptoms. Acceptable forms of chemotherapy, include oral chlorambucil, fludarabine, cladribine, and rituximab. All of these agents have similar activity in WM, with response rates from 40 to 90% in untreated patients. Patients with symptomatic hyperviscosity should be treated with plasmapheresis. Prognostic models have consistently demonstrated that advanced age, cytopenia, hypoalbuminemia, and an elevated β_2-microglobulin are associated with a reduced survival rate.

The present patient was found to have a normal plasma viscosity, normal serum albumin, and normal β_2-microglobulin level. Because he was asymptomatic at diagnosis, a strategy of expectant observation was employed. At 8 months following diagnosis, the patient's IgM level remains stable at 3500 mg/dL.

Clinical Pearls

1. Waldenström's macroglobulinemia (WM) is a low-grade neoplasm of lymphocytic and plasmacytic cells that secrete a monoclonal immunoglobulin M (IgM).

2. Unlike multiple myeloma, lytic bone lesions are typically absent.

3. Hyperviscosity occurs in 15% of patients and is clinically characterized by epistaxis, retinal hemorrhage, and headache. A diagnosis of symptomatic hyperviscosity should be treated with plasmapheresis.

4. Treatment is indicated for patients with anemia, symptoms of hyperviscosity, lymphadenopathy, hepatosplenomegaly, bleeding, or neurological problems. Acceptable forms of chemotherapy include oral chlorambucil, fludarabine, cladribine, and rituximab.

REFERENCES

1. Dimopoulos MA, Panayiotidis P, Moulopoulos LA, et al: Waldenstrom's macroglobulinemia: Clinical features, complications and management. J Clin Oncol 18:214-226, 2000.
2. Raje N, Ferry JA: A 50-year-old man with marked splenomegaly and anemia. N Engl J Med 345:682-687, 2001.
3. Ghobrial IM, Gertz MA, Fonseca R: Waldenstrom's macroglobulinemia. Lancet Oncol 4:679-684, 2003.

PATIENT 11

A 53-year-old woman with fever and diffuse lymphadenopathy after bone marrow transplant

A 53-year-old woman presents with fever to 38.5°C, sore throat, and pruritus of 4-day duration. She underwent a nonmyeloablative peripheral blood stem cell transplant from her sister 88 days before, as treatment for relapsed Hodgkin's lymphoma. She reports no cough, abdominal pain, diarrhea, or dysuria. Her past medical history is significant for retinal detachment and herpes simplex.

Physical Examination: Temperature 38.5°C, blood pressure 110/60 mmHg, pulse 120, Karnofsky Performance Status 90%. General: ill-appearing. HEENT: anicteric sclera, white exudate over tonsils. Lymph nodes: bilateral cervical, axillary, and inguinal lymphadenopathy, less than 2 cm in diameter. Cardiovascular: tachycardic with a soft systolic ejection murmur. Chest: clear to auscultation bilaterally. Abdomen: soft, nontender, normal bowel sounds, without masses or organomegaly. Extremities: no edema. Skin: no rash. Neurological: nonfocal.

Laboratory Findings: Hemoglobin 8.1 g/dL, normal RBC morphology; platelets 429,000/µL; WBC 8400/µL with 53% neutrophils, 21% lymphocytes, 5% monocytes, 11% eosinophils, and 1% basophils. Comprehensive metabolic panel: within normal limits, except albumin 3.3 g/dL. LDH: elevated (233). Blood and urine cultures: negative for 48 hours. Nasopharyngeal swab direct exam: negative for adenovirus, influenza virus types A and B, parainfluenza virus types 1, 2, and 3, and respiratory syncytial virus. Polymerase chain reaction (PCR): strongly positive for Epstein-Barr virus at 6,100,000 copies. Axillary lymph node biopsy: replacement of normal follicular architecture with a pleomorphic lymphoid infiltrate.

Questions: What is the most likely diagnosis? How should this patient be managed? Would the management be different if she were a solid organ transplant recipient?

Answers: Epstein-Barr virus–associated lymphoproliferative disorder is the most likely diagnosis. Anti-CD20 antibodies and donor 1-lymphocyte infusions are commonly used in this setting. In the case of solid organ transplants, decreasing the level of immunosuppression is also an option.

Discussion: Epstein-Barr virus–associated lymphoproliferative disorders (EBV-LPD) are seen following hematopoietic stem cell and solid-organ transplantation and are thought to be associated with the immunosuppression experienced by these patients, specifically, an inadequate cellular immunity against EBV. The term refers to a heterogeneous group of disorders that encompasses polyclonal and oligoclonal B-cell proliferations and monoclonal B-cell lymphomas.

Infection with EBV is very common, with positive serology for the virus being detected in more than 95% of the adult population. If the infection occurs during childhood, it is usually almost asymptomatic. However, if it takes place during adolescence or early adulthood, it frequently presents with an infectious mononucleosis picture, which includes fever, pharyngitis, generalized lymphadenopathy, splenomegaly, and malaise. After replicating in the oropharyngeal mucosa, which serves as the portal of entry, the virus gains access to the bloodstream, where it infects and transforms B-lymphocytes. These transformed B-cells are highly immunogenic and evoke a strong response from cytotoxic T-lymphocytes (CTLs) that, ultimately, are responsible for destruction of the infected B-cells. Some of the infected B-cells, however, express low levels of a restricted number of EBV proteins and are less immunogenic, acting as a reservoir for EBV in the body. During an infected individual's lifespan, it is believed that the virus may reactivate with reinfection of B-cells, but this process is kept under control by EBV-specific CTLs that were generated during the primary response against the virus. However, if that individual's cellular immunity is compromised, as it occurs after transplant, the infectious process may go unchecked and give rise to a lymphoproliferative disorder.

The clinical presentation of post-transplant LPD in hematopoietic stem cell transplant (HSCT) recipients is usually similar to that of infectious mononucleosis, with fever, progressive lymphadenopathy, and pharyngeal exudate. In addition, lymphoproliferative lesions are often found extranodally involving the spleen, liver, lungs, gut, kidneys, and central nervous system. Biopsy is usually needed to establish the diagnosis, and EBV products can be detected by *in situ* hybridization. Analysis of immunoglobulin gene rearrangement patterns or of the presence of fused termini of the EBV genome in the cells can be used to demonstrate clonality. Also, in the HSCT setting, cytogenetic or molecular testing demonstrates that, in the majority of cases, the malignant cells are from donor origin. Detection of Epstein-Barr virus DNA by PCR in the peripheral blood of affected patients can also be used to support the diagnosis.

The overall incidence of post-transplant LPD in recipients of HSCT is 1% at 10 years, but the risk varies according to the source and preparation of stem cells. T-cell depleted grafts, unrelated or human leukocyte antigen–mismatched grafts, and the use of anti-thymocyte globulin for graft versus host disease prophylaxis each increase the relative risk of developing the condition. The peak incidence occurs during the first 6 to 12 months post-transplant. Monoclonal disease was traditionally refractory to treatment until the development of two therapeutic interventions: adoptive transfer of CTLs and monoclonal anti-B-cell antibodies.

Because the malignant B-clone is derived from cells harvested from donors who have no evidence of LPD, a few years ago it was reasoned that the transfer of lymphocytes collected from the HSC donor might restore the immunological balance by providing enough EBV-specific CTLs. Indeed, patients with post-HSCT lymphoproliferative disorders were effectively treated after receiving unmanipulated donor T-cells (donor lymphocyte infusions). Because the T-cells infused are likely to contain alloreactive, non–EBV-specific lymphocytes, there is a chance of inducing GVHD. Because of this issue, a number of methods have been proposed to develop and select in vitro donor CTLs that are specific for EBV epitopes, prior to administering them to patients with lymphoproliferative disorder. These EBV-specific CTLs have been used with success in the treatment and prophylaxis of LPD in a small number of patients. A disadvantage of these methods compared to unmodified donor lymphocyte infusions is that they are quite labor intensive and require considerable amount of time to be generated.

The availability of monoclonal anti-B-cell antibodies has also been quite promising. Several small studies have shown that administration of a monoclonal anti-CD20 antibody (rituximab) can induce complete remissions in a significant proportion of patients. Furthermore, rituximab has been used for prophylaxis and preemptive treatment of EBV-LPD.

Contrary to the case of HSCT, malignant clones arising in the post solid-organ transplant setting are derived from recipient lymphocytes. Primary infection after transplant (transmitted by donor B-cells within the graft) and increased levels of immunosuppression are the main risk factors for developing LPD after solid-organ transplantation. Because a decrease in the degree of immunosuppression can restore some of the competence against EBV-derived tumors, reduction or withdrawal of immunosuppression is often used as first line of therapy. However, care must be used when rejection of the transplanted organ, a likely consequence of this intervention, may be fatal. Chemotherapy as well as immunotherapy with IFN-α has been used to treat post solid-organ transplant LPD, but results are not uniform. Once again, monoclonal anti-B-cell antibodies have had promising results. Moreover, the use of host derived EBV-specific CTLs is being currently investigated.

The present patient received a combination of donor lymphocyte infusions and rituximab, which she tolerated well. The lymphadenopathy resolved and her peripheral blood EBV-PCR became negative. She is being closely watched for Hodgkin's disease recurrence.

Clinical Pearls

1. Epstein-Barr virus–associated lymphoproliferative disorders (EBV-LPDs) are due to impaired cellular immunity against EBV occurring after hematopoietic stem cell transplant (HSCT) and its conditioning regimens, or related to immunosuppressive drugs used after solid-organ transplants.

2. The clinical manifestations are similar to the infectious mononucleosis syndrome.

3. The malignant cell in monoclonal EBV-LPDs is a B-lymphocyte of donor origin in cases associated with HSCT, whereas it is of host origin in those related to solid-organ transplant.

4. Anti-CD20 antibodies and cytotoxic T-lymphocytes, EBV-specific or not, are the most promising therapies for monoclonal EBV-LPD.

REFERENCES

1. Papadopoulos EB, Ladanyi M, Emanuel D, et al: Infusions of donor leukocytes to treat Epstein-Barr virus-associated lymphoproliferative disorders after allogeneic bone marrow transplantation. N Engl J Med 330:1185-1191, 1994.
2. Faye A, Quartier P, Reguerre Y, et al: Chimaeric anti-CD20 monoclonal antibody (rituximab) in post-transplant B-lymphoproliferative disorder following stem cell transplantation in children. Br J Haematol 115:112-118, 2001.
3. Straathof KC, Bollard CM, Rooney CM, et al: Immunotherapy for Epstein-Barr virus-associated cancers in children. Oncologist 8:83-98, 2003.

PATIENT 12

A 70-year-old smoker with shortness of breath and weight loss

A 70-year-old man presents with shortness of breath, nonproductive cough, chest pain for 2 weeks, and a 20-pound weight loss. He denies dysphagia, hemoptysis, and night sweats. He reports smoking 1.5 packs of cigarettes per day for 40 years.

Physical Examination: General: appears fatigued; mild respiratory distress. Temperature 37.3°C, blood pressure 96/64 mmHg, pulse 110, oxygen saturation (pulse oximetry) 94% at rest on 3 L oxygen. HEENT: anicteric, palpable left supraclavicular and left submandibular lymph nodes. Chest: decreased breath sounds and dullness to percussion at the left lung base. Cardiac: tachycardic, no murmur or rub.

Laboratory Findings: CBC: normal. Sodium 129, potassium 4.7, creatinine 1.4. Transaminases: normal. CT scan of chest: left hilar mass measuring 6.5 cm × 2.3 cm encasing left main pulmonary artery, moderate-sized left pleural effusion, multiple left pulmonary nodules (see Figures). Pathology: fine-needle aspiration of left supraclavicular node, positive for small cell carcinoma.

Questions: What is this patient's diagnosis and clinical stage? What are the treatment options?

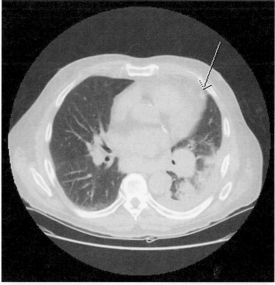

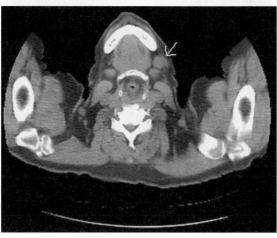

Answers: This patient has "extensive-stage" small cell lung cancer. The recommended treatment is combination chemotherapy.

Discussion: Small cell lung cancer represents 15 to 25% of diagnosed lung cancers. This disease is characterized by its rapid doubling time, high growth fraction, and early development of metastasis. Because of its aggressive clinical course, without treatment the median survival from time of diagnosis is 2 to 4 months.

Small cell lung cancer tends to be more widely disseminated at the time of diagnosis compared to other types of lung cancer. For staging simplicity, extent of disease is usually classified as "limited stage" or "extensive stage." The TNM system is less commonly used. At the time of diagnosis, 25 to 30% of patients are limited stage, defined as disease restricted to the hemithorax of origin, mediastinum, or supraclavicular lymph nodes (located within a single radiotherapy port). With treatment, median survival for limited stage disease is 16 to 24 months.

Small cell lung cancer that has spread beyond the supraclavicular areas (beyond a single radiation port) is classified as extensive stage, and is associated with worse prognosis. Presence of malignant pleural effusion also classifies patients as extensive stage, as in this case. Median survival in extensive stage disease is 6 to 12 months with therapy, with fewer than 5% of patients surviving for 2 years. Patients present with extensive disease 70 to 75% of the time.

Combination chemotherapy is the standard of care for extensive-stage small cell lung cancer, with two or more drugs required to achieve maximal benefit. Response rates are high (70-85%), with complete responses in 20 to 30% of patients. Unfortunately, despite initial chemosensitivity, prolonged responses are rare. Multiple combination regimens have been evaluated, with similar reported efficacy. Standard combination regimens include etoposide plus cisplatin (EP), etoposide plus carboplatin (EC), or regimens containing irinotecan (such as cisplatin plus irinotecan). Other regimens include CAV (cyclophosphamide, doxorubicin, vincristine), CAE (cyclophosphamide, doxorubicin, etoposide), and ICE (ifosfamide, carboplatin, etoposide). There appears to be no role for maintenance chemotherapy beyond four to six cycles, with minor prolongation of response and no survival benefit. The addition of chest irradiation to chemotherapy does not appear to improve survival in patients with extensive-stage disease, although it may be warranted for symptom control.

Pretreatment features associated with prolonged survival include good performance status, female gender, and limited-stage disease. Central nervous system or liver involvement at diagnosis predicts worse outcome.

Prophylactic cranial irradiation (PCI) can be considered in patients with extensive-stage disease who have achieved a complete remission with chemotherapy. There is a greater than 60% risk of developing brain metastases, and this may be reduced by 50% with PCI. Although PCI has a more clear role in patients with limited-stage disease when the goal is long-term remission, the true benefit in patients with extensive-stage disease is not as well known because these patients are just as likely to progress in other metastatic sites. Radiotherapy to other areas is reserved for symptom palliation (e.g., bony metastases or persistent superior vena cava syndrome).

Paraneoplastic syndromes may occur, with endocrine (SIADH, ectopic ACTH syndrome) or neurological (antibody-mediated) manifestations. In this patient with hyponatremia, measurement of urine electrolytes to evaluate for the presence of SIADH should be undertaken. SIADH is a poor prognostic sign in small cell lung cancer and should be managed by fluid restriction in mild cases, or with hypertonic saline in more severe cases. Demeclocycline, an antibiotic that induces a counteracting nephrogenic diabetes insipidus, can also be prescribed in more severe or refractory situations. The overall management, however, requires treatment of the underlying malignancy.

In the present patient, further workup revealed multiple brain lesions. He therefore underwent palliative whole brain irradiation, followed by combination chemotherapy with EC, a regimen chosen due to multiple comorbidities.

Clinical Pearls

1. Small cell lung cancer is classified as "limited stage" (within a single radiotherapy port) or "extensive stage."

2. In extensive-stage disease, combination chemotherapy prolongs survival. Although small cell cancer is usually chemosensitive, prolonged remissions are rare.

3. Prophylactic cranial irradiation should be considered in patients with extensive-stage disease who have achieved a complete remission with chemotherapy.

REFERENCES

1. Spiro SG, Souhami RL, Geddes DM: Duration of chemotherapy in small cell lung cancer: A Cancer Research Campaign trial. Br J Cancer 59(4):578-583, 1989.
2. Adjei AA, Marks RS, Bonner JA: Current guidelines for the management of small cell lung cancer. Mayo Clin Proc 74(8):809-816, 1999.
3. Auperin A, Arriagada R, Pignon JP, et al: for Prophylactic Cranial Irradiation Overview Collaborative Group: Prophylactic cranial irradiation for patients with small-cell lung cancer in complete remission. N Engl J Med 341(7):476-484, 1999.
4. Paesmans M, Sculier JP, Lecomte J: Prognostic factors for patients with small cell lung carcinoma: Analysis of a series of 763 patients included in four consecutive prospective trials with a minimum follow-up of 5 years. Cancer 89:523-533, 2000.
5. Noda K, Nishiwaki Y, Kawahara M: Irinotecan plus cisplatin compared with etoposide plus cisplatin for extensive small-cell lung cancer. N Engl J Med 346:85-91, 2002.
6. Simon GR, Wagner H: for American College of Chest Physicians: Small cell lung cancer. Chest 123(1 Suppl):259S-271S, 2003.

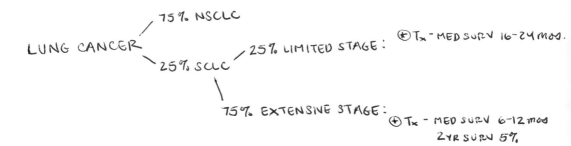

LUNG CANCER
- 75% NSCLC
- 25% SCLC
  - 25% LIMITED STAGE: (+)Tx - MED SURV 16-24 mos.
  - 75% EXTENSIVE STAGE: (+)Tx - MED SURV 6-12 mos
    2YR SURV 5%

- φTx, MED SURV. 2-4mos FROM Dx

- FOR ES SCLC, NO ROLE FOR XRT OUTSIDE OF PALLIATION

- GOOD Px FACTORS: GOOD PS, ♀, LS SCLC
  POOR Px FACTORS: CNS/LIVER INVOLVEMENT

- RISK FOR BRAIN METS 60% IN ES SCLC. CAN ↓ TO 30% W/ PCI.

PATIENT 13

A 68-year-old man with multiple colonic polyps found on routine colonoscopy

A 68-year-old man with a past medical history significant for diabetes and hypertension presents to his gastroenterologist for a routine screening colonoscopy. The patient denies rectal bleeding, constipation, diarrhea, and weight loss. At colonoscopy he is found to have multiple polyps throughout his colon.

Physical Examination: General: well-appearing. Vitals: stable. HEENT: no pallor or icterus. Lymph nodes: no palpable peripheral adenopathy. Cardiac: regular rate and rhythm. Chest: clear to auscultation bilaterally. Abdomen: soft, nontender, no hepatosplenomegaly. Extremities: normal.

Laboratory Findings: Hemoglobin: 10.3 g/dL, platelets 183,000/µL, WBC 7500/µL. Chemistry panel: normal. CT abdomen: no abnormality detected. Colonic biopsy: diffuse atypical lymphoid infiltration. Lymphoid cells stain positively for CD19, CD20, and CD5 and negatively for CD10 and CD23.

Questions: What is the most likely diagnosis? What additional stain will help confirm this patient's diagnosis?

Answers: Mantle cell lymphoma (lymphomatous polyposis) is the likely diagnosis, and a positive stain for cyclin D1 will confirm this.

Discussion: Mantle cell lymphoma (MCL) is a relatively uncommon type of non-Hodgkin's lymphoma accounting for approximately 5% of all lymphomas in the United States. MCL is a unique clinicopathological entity with distinct morphological, immunophenotypic, cytogenetic, and molecular characteristics.

Clinically, MCL is considered an intermediate-grade lymphoma. The median age at presentation is 58, and there is a marked male predominance. Advanced stage at presentation is typical, with bone marrow and peripheral blood involvement commonly seen. Splenomegaly is detected in 30 to 60% of patients. Extranodal sites are frequently involved, including Waldeyer's ring, liver, the central nervous system, and a peculiar predilection for gastrointestinal (GI) involvement (up to 80% in some series). This may present as a distinctive syndrome of multiple lymphomatous polyposis of the large bowel, as illustrated by this patient. B-symptoms are present in 30 to 60% of patients. Elevated LDH and β_2-microglobulin are detected in 50% of cases.

Four distinct histological subtypes of MCL are recognized: mantle-zone pattern, nodular subtype, diffuse subtype, and blastoid variant. The mantle-zone variant is generally considered to have a more benign clinical course; the blastoid variant is considered the most aggressive and is associated with a poorer prognosis.

The immunophenotype of MCL is of a B-cell disorder expressing CD19, CD20, and CD22. A peculiar characteristic of MCL, similar to chronic lymphocytic leukemia/small lymphocytic lymphoma (CLL/SLL), is the coexpression of the T-cell–associated antigen CD5 in almost all cases. Morphologically similar, the salient features that distinguish MCL from CLL/SLL are the expression of cyclin D1 and FMC-7 and a lack of CD23 expression. CD23 is expressed in virtually all cases of CLL/SLL. Overexpression of cyclin D1 is a constant and specific finding in MCL. Another distinguishing feature of MCL that allows distinction from CLL/SLL is moderate to strong intensity of surface immunoglobulin staining in MCL and dim surface immunoglobulin (Ig) staining in CLL/SLL. Virtually all cases of MCL carry the t(11;14) (q13:q32) cytogenetic alteration on karyotype analysis or FISH. This reciprocal translocation juxtaposes the immunoglobulin heavy chain locus and the cyclin D1 gene.

In contrast to CLL/SLL, the clinical course of MCL is relatively aggressive, with poor response to conventional therapeutic regimens. Responses to chemotherapy, such as cyclophosphamide, hydroxydaunomycin, Oncovin, plus prednisone (CHOP) or cyclophosphamide, vincristine, plus (CVP) are usually only partial, and even in cases achieving complete remission, the duration of remission is usually short. Autologous transplantation has not proven curative. The median survival in most published series is approximately 3 to 4 years. The clinical parameters associated with poor prognosis include advanced age, poor performance status, advanced stage, splenomegaly, peripheral blood involvement, high LDH, low serum albumin, and anemia. Surprisingly, the international prognostic index is not of consistent prognostic value. The architectural pattern of nodal involvement is of some predictive value, with the mantle-zone pattern associated with a higher proportion of complete remissions and longer survival. In contrast, the blastic variants have an aggressive course characterized by failure to obtain complete remission and a short median survival of approximately 18 months.

Recently, researchers at the MD Anderson Cancer Center have reported their phase II experience with the hyper-CVAD regimen for the treatment of MCL. This regimen includes hyperfractionated cyclophosphamide, vincristine, doxorubicin, and dexamethasone, which is given alternately with high doses of cytarabine and methotrexate and leucovorin rescue therapy. After four to six courses, this is followed by consolidation with high-dose cyclophosphamide and total body irradiation in patients younger than 65 years. At 3 years the overall survival and event-free survival rates were 92% and 72%, respectively, for previously untreated patients. The event-free survival (EFS) of 72% compares favorably to the 28% EFS in a historical control group who received CHOP or a CHOP-like regimen. More recently, these researchers have incorporated rituximab to the hyper-CVAD regimen, with promising early results. Single-agent rituximab has an objective response rate of approximately 30% in MCL. Other promising investigational approaches include radioimmunotherapy and nonmyeloablative stem cell transplantation. Enrollment on a clinical trial is the current best therapeutic recommendation in this disease, where there is no standard approach and no clear curative strategy.

The present patient was treated on an experimental protocol, with radioimmunotherapy and chemotherapy. At the end of treatment, a repeat colonic biopsy revealed persistent cecal involvement with MCL. The patient, subsequently, received a purine analog in combination with cyclophosphamide and rituximab, achieving a complete remission. He remains in remission 6 months after completing all therapy.

Clinical Pearls

1. The immunophenotype of MCL is of a B-cell disorder expressing CD19, CD20, and CD22. Coexpression of the T-cell–associated antigen CD5 and cyclin D1 is seen in almost all cases.

2. Virtually all cases of MCL carry the t(11;14) (q13:q32) cytogenetic alteration on karyotype analysis or FISH.

3. In contrast to CLL/SLL, the clinical course of MCL is relatively aggressive with poor response to conventional therapeutic regimens. Responses to chemotherapy, such as CHOP or CVP, are usually only partial; even in cases achieving complete remission, the duration of remission is usually short.

REFERENCES

1. Argatoff LH, Connors JM, Klasa RJ, et al: Mantle cell lymphoma: A clinicopathologic study of 80 cases. Blood 89(6):2067-2078, 1997.
2. Campo E, Raffeld M, Jaffe ES: Mantle cell lymphoma. Semin Hematol 36(2):115-127, 1999.
3. Press O: Treatment of mantle-cell lymphoma: Stem cell transplantation, radioimmunotherapy, and management of mantle-cell lymphoma subsets. American Society of Clinical Oncology Educational Book, 2002.

PATIENT 14

A 31-year-old woman with right-sided neck swelling

A 31-year-old woman began to notice mild right-sided neck swelling 2 years ago. During the month prior to presentation, the swelling has markedly increased. The patient has no significant past medical history. She has not experienced fevers, night sweats, or weight loss.

Physical Examination: Temperature 36.6°C, heart rate 80, blood pressure 120/80 mmHg, respirations 16, weight 70.9 kg. General: well-appearing. HEENT: pupils equal, round, and reactive to light; sclera anicteric; oropharynx clear. Lymph nodes: multiple, greater than 2-cm anterior cervical lymph nodes from angle of jaw to above clavicle. No other cervical, axillary, or inguinal lymphadenopathy. Chest: clear. Cardiovascular: regular rate and rhythm, no murmurs. Abdomen: soft, nontender, no distention, no hepatosplenomegaly. Extremities: no edema.

Laboratory Findings: WBC 8700/μL, hemoglobin 12.6 g/dL, platelets 267/μL. Biochemistry profile: electrolytes normal. BUN 20 mg/dL, creatinine 0.9 mg/dL. Liver function tests: AST 14, ALT 17, albumin 4.5 g/dL, total bilirubin 0.5 mg/dL, lactate dehydrogenase 151. Erythrocyte sedimentation rate: 46 mm/hr. CT scan of chest, abdomen, and pelvis: right-sided lymphadenopathy, 5 cm in AP diameter. PET scan: significant for increased uptake in internal jugular chain and spinal accessory chain on right as well as in left supraclavicular region. Fine-needle aspiration of a right cervical lymph node: CD15/CD30–positive cells scattered among a background of large lymphocytes.

Questions: What is the diagnosis? What are the risks of combined modality therapy for this patient?

Answers: Stage I (early-stage) Hodgkin's disease is the diagnosis. The radiation component of combined modality therapy involves risk of late toxicity.

Discussion: Approximately 7500 diagnoses of Hodgkin's disease are made in the United States annually. It is most commonly a disease of the young, with the highest incidence occurring in patients between ages 15 and 30. Hodgkin's disease is a potentially curable illness; approximately 80 to 85% of patients achieve long-term survival. Survival for early-stage disease is over 90%. With such a high number of long-term survivors, identifying the minimal curative therapy with the least long-term toxicity has become paramount. The staging of Hodgkin's disease is based on the modified Ann Arbor staging system. Treatment for Hodgkin's disease is based on stage and specific prognostic factors. Early-stage Hodgkin's disease is classified as stages I and IIA. Patients with early-stage disease and a favorable prognosis do not have any of the following criteria: bulky mediastinal disease, an elevated erythrocyte sedimentation rate, three or more involved lymph node areas, extranodal disease, B-symptoms, or age greater than 50 at diagnosis.

Historically, primary extended field irradiation was the treatment of choice for early-stage Hodgkin's disease. A high relapse rate and recognition of fatal long-term complications secondary to mediastinal radiation has led to a markedly decreased use of this single treatment modality. Long-term side effects of radiation therapy include secondary malignancies, cardiac disease, pulmonary fibrosis, thyroid dysfunction, and fatigue. Patients who were treated with radiation therapy have a continuously increasing risk of developing a secondary solid tumor throughout their lives. The risk of leukemia seems to plateau at 15 years. In one of the largest studies of long-term survivors, approximately 26% of patients developed a secondary solid tumor by 30 years. Many patients developed multiple malignancies and at ages younger than the general population.

Currently, combined modality therapy with *chemotherapy* and *involved field radiation therapy* is being used for patients with favorable early-stage disease. Involved field radiation is administered after successful chemotherapy. There is no advantage to more extended radiation therapy fields. The standard chemotherapy regimen comprises doxorubicin, bleomycin, vinblastine, and dacarbazine (ABVD) for four cycles (eight treatments), followed by 30 to 35 Gy of involved field irradiation. Overall survival at 10 years has not been shown to be different between combined modality therapy and primary extended field radiation therapy alone. Clinical trials are underway to evaluate the benefit of treatment with chemotherapy alone in early-stage disease. The first randomized trial to compare ABVD chemotherapy with ABVD chemotherapy and radiation therapy has recently been completed. There was no statistically significant difference found in overall survival between the two groups. However, the median duration of follow-up was less than 5 years. Studies evaluating overall survival of patients at 10, 20, or more years are still needed before a conclusion can be made regarding the benefit of single modality chemotherapy in favorable early-stage Hodgkin's disease.

The present patient began treatment with ABVD chemotherapy. She opted to not have radiation therapy because of the risk of late toxicity and the lack of increase in survival.

Clinical Pearls

1. Treatment of patients with Hodgkin's disease depends on staging and prognostic factors.

2. Favorable early-stage disease patients should be treated with doxorubicin, bleomycin, vinblastine, and dacarbazine (ABVD)) and involved field radiation therapy. ABVD alone may be considered in select circumstances.

3. Potential late toxicities of radiation therapy must be fully explained to the patient; monitoring for secondary effects is an important component of care for the patient with Hodgkin's disease.

REFERENCES

1. Specht L, Gray RG, Clarke MJ, Peto R: Influence of more extensive radiotherapy and adjuvant chemotherapy on long-term outcome of early-stage Hodgkin's disease: A meta-analysis of 23 randomized trials involving 3888 patients. International Hodgkin's Disease Collaborative Group. J Clin Oncol 16:830-843, 1998.
2. Dores G, Curtis R, Travis L: Second cancer risk following Hodgkin's disease: Analysis of 15,465 patients reported to the National Cancer Institute's Surveillance, Epidemiology and End Results (SEER) program. Proc Am Soc Clin Oncol 1127a, 2001.
3. Ekstrand BC, Horning SJ: Hodgkin's disease. Blood Rev 16:111-117, 2002.
4. Diehl V, Stein H, Hummel M, et al: Hodgkin's Lymphoma: Biology and Treatment Strategies for Primary, Refractory and Relapsed Disease. American Society of Hematology Education Book, Jan 2003, pp 225-247.
5. Laskar S, Gupta T, Vimal S, et al: Consolidation radiation after complete remission in Hodgkin's disease following six cycles of doxorubicin, bleomycin, vinblastine, and dacarbazine chemotherapy: Is there a need? J Clin Oncol 22(1):62-68, 2004.

PATIENT 15

A 60-year-old man with diffuse lymphadenopathy

A 60-year-old man with bilateral axillary swelling of 2-year duration presents with diffuse cervical and inguinal lymphadenopathy on a routine physical examination.

Physical Examination: General: well-appearing. Temperature 36°C, pulse 68, blood pressure 130/90. HEENT: anicteric, no tonsillar enlargement. Cardiac: regular rate and rhythm without murmurs. Chest: clear to auscultation. Abdomen: soft, no hepatosplenomegaly. Extremities: no edema. Lymph nodes: left axillary 2 cm, right axillary 1.5 cm, bilateral cervical and inguinal less than 1 cm.

Laboratory Findings: Hemoglobin: 16 g/dL, WBC 7100/μL, platelets 257,000/μL, mean corpuscular volume 84.7 fl, RDW 12.4%, neutrophils 69%, lymphocytes 23%. Peripheral blood smear: normal. Electrolytes: normal. ESR 1 mm/hr, CRP 0.2, lactate dehydrogenase 146. Heterophile test: negative. Right groin lymph node biopsy: small lymphocytes with nuclear indentations (centrocytes) and larger lymphocytes without indentations (centroblasts; see Figures). Flow cytometry: λ light chain–restricted monoclonal population coexpressing CD10, CD19, CD20, and FMC7.

Questions: What is the most likely diagnosis? What is the appropriate management of this disorder?

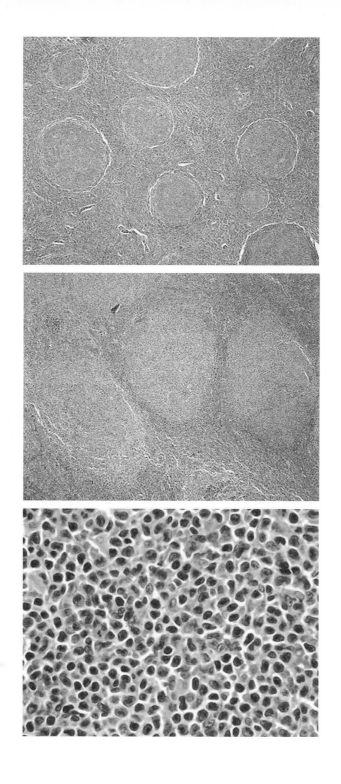

Answers: Follicular lymphoma is the likely diagnosis. The recommended management is observation.

Discussion: Follicular lymphoma (FL) is the most common indolent non-Hodgkin's lymphoma (NHL) and the second most common lymphoma after diffuse large B-cell type (DLBCL). It is of B-cell origin and represents approximately 20% of total lymphoma incidence. Median age at diagnosis is 60 years, with slight female predominance, unlike other NHLs. Follicular lymphomas are more common in the United States and in Europe.

The presentation of this patient is typical of follicular lymphoma, with painless diffuse lymphadenopathy that has been present for a long duration without significant symptoms. B-symptoms, consisting of fever greater than 38°C, drenching night sweats, or weight loss greater than 10%, occur only about 20% of the time. Bone marrow is involved in 60 to 70% of cases, leading to Ann Arbor stage IV in the majority at presentation.

Under the microscope, follicular lymphomas resemble normal germinal centers of secondary lymphoid follicles. They consist of a mixture of centrocytes and centroblasts. The higher the proportion of centroblasts, the higher is the grading and the aggressiveness of the follicular lymphoma. For example, grade III has more than 15 centroblasts per high power field and is actually grouped with aggressive lymphomas because it behaves more like DLBCL. Grade I, which has fewer than five centroblasts, is the most common subtype.

Follicular lymphoma cells express B-cell antigens (CD19, CD20, CD21), CD10, HLA-DR, and surface immunoglobulins; they are negative for CD5 and cyclin D1. The immunoglobulin genes are rearranged, and variable portions have somatic mutations. Cytogenetics show t(14;18) translocation in 85% of cases, juxtaposing Ig heavy chain and bcl-2 oncogene. This translocation confirms FL but cannot be used as the sole basis of diagnosis because it may also be present in normal individuals.

The International Prognostic Index (IPI) that was developed for DLBLC is of lesser utility in FL because only 10% have high-risk IPI scores. An international cooperative study recently proposed a follicular lymphoma international prognostic index (FLIPI), which includes age over 60, Ann Arbor stage III or IV, more than 4 nodal areas of involvement, hemoglobin less than 12, and elevated LDH. Patient with 0/1 risk factors had 10-year overall survival of 70.7%; those with 2 risk factors, 50.9%; and those in a high-risk group with three or more risk factors, 10-year overall survival of 35.5%.

Follicular lymphoma has median survival of over 8 years, with the notable exception of high-risk IPI patients, whose median survival is 1 year. The disease can be characterized as indolent but incurable: It responds well to radiation and chemotherapy but, eventually, relapses. If it transforms to DLBCL, which occurs at the rate of about 5 to 10% a year, the FL often relapses, even if the DLBCL is cured.

The treatment of FL remains controversial. The minority of patients with early-stage (I and II) follicular lymphomas can be treated with regional radiation therapy, administering 30 to 40 Gray to the involved or extended field. This results in a 40% 10-year disease-free survival.

The Stanford experience demonstrates that patients with advanced FL can be observed without compromising their survival. The Groupe d'Etude Lymphomes Folliculaire (GELF) criteria estimate tumor burden and are most often used in deciding to initiate treatment (see Table). Once the decision to treat is made, there are several possible approaches, including single-agent rituximab, or a combination of rituximab with CVP, CEPP, or CHOP; single-agent purine analogs, and radioimmunotherapy could also be used. More aggressive treatments, including autologous transplants, often result in increased disease-free survival but not improved overall survival. Allogeneic transplant is the only potentially curative treatment; it may improve overall survival to about 80% but results in treatment-related mortality of up to 30%. Mortality is improving, however, particularly with advent of non-myeloablative ("mini") allogenic transplantation. Given the lack of curative options, participation in clinical trials is of great importance.

The present patient with at least stage III (bone marrow was not taken), grade 1 follicular lymphoma, accepted a trial of observation. He has been followed uneventfully for 9 months.

GELF Criteria for High Tumor Burden in Follicular Lymphoma

Systemic symptoms
Three or more lymph nodes sites > 3 cm
   in diameter
A single lymph node site > 7 cm in diameter
Platelets < 100,000/μL or absolute
   neutrophil count < 1000/μL
Circulating lymphoma cells > 5000/μL
Marked splenomegaly, compressive
   symptoms, pleural effusion, or ascites

Clinical Pearls

1. Follicular lymphoma (FL) is the most common indolent non-Hodgkin's lymphoma.

2. Under the microscope, follicular lymphoma resembles germinal centers of lymphoid follicles.

3. Follicular lymphoma cells stain for HLA-DR, CD19, CD20, CD21, and usually for CD10 and surface immunoglobulin; have rearranged immunoglobulin genes; and often have the t(14;18) translocation.

4. Management of FL is controversial. Some cases of early FL can be treated with radiation. An initial trial of observation is acceptable.

REFERENCES

1. Solal-Celigny P, Roy P, Colombat P, et al: Follicular Lymphoma International Prognostic Index. Blood 104(5):1258-1265, 2004.
2. Brice P, Bastion Y, Lepage E, et al: Comparison in low-tumor-burden follicular lymphomas between an initial no-treatment policy, prednimustine, or interferon alpha: A randomized study from the Groupe d'Etude des Lymphomes Folliculaires. Groupe d'Etude des Lymphomes de l'Adulte. J Clin Oncol 15(3):1110-1117, 1997.
3. Mac Manus MP, Hoppe RT: Is radiotherapy curative for stages I and II low-grade follicular lymphoma? Results of a long-term follow-up study of patients treated at Stanford University. J Clin Oncol 14(4):1282-1290, 1996.
4. Horning SJ, Rosenberg SA: The natural history of initially untreated low-grade non-Hodgkin's lymphomas. N Engl J Med 311(23):1471-1475, 1984.
5. Portlock CS, Rosenberg SA: No initial therapy for stage III and IV non-Hodgkin's lymphomas of favorable histologic types. Ann Intern Med 90(1):10-13, 1979.

PATIENT 16

A 56-year-old woman with an elevated hematocrit and pruritus

A 56-year-old woman with a past medical history significant for early-stage breast cancer presents to her physician, complaining of pruritus after warm showers. She denies experiencing headaches or change in vision. She denies any tobacco use.

Physical Examination: General: well-appearing, thin, plethoric. Vital signs: stable. Oxygen saturation: 98% on room air. HEENT: unremarkable. Nodes: no palpable adenopathy. Heart: regular rate and rhythm. Chest: clear to auscultation bilaterally. Abdomen: firm, tender spleen tip palpable 3 cm below left costal margin. Extremities: no clubbing, cyanosis, or edema.

Laboratory Findings: CBC: hematocrit 58%, WBC 15,000/μL, platelets 485,000/μL. Biochemistry profile: normal. ^{51}Cr-labeled red blood cell mass study: elevated red blood cell mass and normal plasma volume.

Questions: What additional studies are required to confirm this woman's diagnosis? What would be the initial therapeutic recommendation?

Answers: Serum erythropoietin level will help establish the diagnosis of polycythemia vera. Initial treatment should include therapeutic phlebotomy and aspirin.

Discussion: Polycythemia vera (PV) is a neoplastic disorder originating from a hematopoietic stem cell, resulting in the overproduction of red blood cells. It is characterized by an *elevated red cell mass* in the absence of conditions that induce secondary polycythemia.

At presentation most patients with PV have symptoms. Headache, weakness, and pruritus after bathing in hot water are particularly frequent complaints. One third of patients describe visual changes, weight loss, epigastric pain, excessive sweating, and/or painful paresthesias of the hands and feet (erythromelalgia). Up to 20% of patients present with a large-vessel thrombotic complication, such as a cerebrovascular accident, myocardial infarction, deep venous thrombosis, or hepatic vein thrombosis. Clinical signs at diagnosis include splenomegaly, plethora, and hypertension.

An elevated hematocrit may result from either an increase in the total red cell mass (RCM) or a decrease in total plasma volume. An isolated decrease in plasma volume is termed *relative* or *apparent* polycythemia and is also known as *Gaisböck's syndrome.* The most common causes for relative polycythemia include diuretic and alcohol use.

Obtaining an RCM is the first step in evaluating a patient with an elevated hematocrit. This is performed by labeling a sample of the patient's blood with ^{51}CR prior to reinfusion. A second sample is then drawn from the patient to determine the concentration of ^{51}CR-labeled RBCs. In parallel ^{125}I-labeled albumin is injected to assess the plasma volume. A diagnosis of absolute erythrocytosis is made when an individual's measured RCM is more than 25% above the mean predicted value.

After confirmation of an elevated RCM, additional studies are required to differentiate PV from *secondary polycythemia* (see Table 1). In PV, *erythropoietin (EPO) levels* are typically low. In contrast, most acquired secondary causes of polycythemia are associated with elevated or high/normal EPO levels. Other studies to determine the cause of a secondary polycythemia should include a thorough history (including tobacco history and symptoms of obstructive sleep apnea); careful physical examination; arterial oxygen saturation; carbon-monoxy hemoglobin level; ferritin, vitamin B_{12}, and folate levels; renal function; hepatic function tests; abdominal ultrasound; sleep study; pulmonary function testing; chest X-ray; and oxygen dissociation curve (to identify patients with high oxygen affinity Hb and rare patients with con-

Table 1. Common Causes of Secondary Erythrocytosis

Congenital
   Mutant high oxygen affinity hemoglobin
   Congenital low 2,3-DPG
Acquired
   Arterial hypoxemia
      Cyanotic congenital heart disease
      Chronic pulmonary disease
      Smoking
   Renal lesions
      Renal cell cancer
      Renal cysts
      Hydronephrosis
      Renal artery stenosis
   Hepatic lesions
      Hepatocellular carcinoma
      Cirrhosis
      Hepatitis
   Drugs
      Androgens
   Endocrine tumors
      Adrenal tumors
   Miscellaneous tumors
      Cerebellar hemangioblastoma
      Uterine fibroids
      Bronchial carcinoma

DPG = diphosphoglycerate.

genitally low 2,3-diphosphoglycerate levels), as clinically indicated.

In the absence of causes for secondary polycythemia, and with a low EPO level, polycythemia vera is the most likely diagnosis. Clinical criteria to standardize the diagnosis for patients on treatment protocols have been established (see Table 2).

PV is a chronic disease that is incurable with conventional therapy. The clinical course is characterized by a significant risk of thrombotic complications and variable risk of transformation to myeloid metaplasia with myelofibrosis or acute myeloid. Untreated patients have a median survival of 18 months because of the high incidence of fatal thrombotic events. Cytoreductive therapy, using phlebotomy or chemotherapy, reduces the incidence of thrombotic events and significantly improves survival. The goals of treatment are to minimize the risk of thrombotic complications and to prevent progression to myelofibrosis or leukemia.

Therapeutic phlebotomy, removing 500 mL of blood weekly until a hematocrit of 40 to 45% is achieved, has become standard. Serial phlebotomy

Table 2. Diagnostic Criteria for Polycythemia Vera

A1	Raised RCM (> 25% above normal predicted value)
A2	Absence of causes of secondary polycythemia
A3	Palpable splenomegaly
A4	Clonality marker (abnormal marrow karyotype)
B1	Thrombocytosis (platelet count > 400,000/μL)
B2	Neutrophil leukocytosis (neutrophil count > 10,000/μL or > 12,500/μL in smokers)
B3	Splenomegaly demonstrated by isotope or ultrasound scanning
B4	Endogenous erythroid colony growth or low serum EPO level

RCM = total red cell mass; EPO = erythropoietin.
A1 + A2 + A3 or A4 establishes the diagnosis.
A1 + A2 + two of B establishes the diagnosis.

will result in the development of iron deficiency, limiting the patient's ability to make red blood cells. Patients should not take iron-containing multivitamins. Care must be taken in phlebotomy not to make the patient truly iron deficient because it may lead to a reactive thrombocytosis and it increases the risk of thrombosis. Patients managed by phlebotomy alone have an increased risk of thrombosis during the first 3 years after initiation of therapy.

Based on this observation, patients who have had a prior thrombotic event, or who are older than 60 years, should probably be treated with phlebotomy and a myelosuppressive agent as initial treatment. The efficacy and safety of antithrombotic drugs in patients with polycythemia vera are uncertain. Aspirin has been long avoided because a trial conducted by the Polycythemia Vera Study Group reported a high incidence of gastrointestinal bleeding in patients who received a high dose of aspirin (900 mg daily). Recently, however, a double-blind, placebo-controlled, randomized trial to assess the safety and efficacy of prophylaxis with low-dose aspirin (100 mg daily) has been reported. In this study of over 500 patients, treatment with aspirin, as compared with placebo, reduced the risk of the combined end point of nonfatal myocardial infarction, nonfatal stroke, and death from cardiovascular causes. The incidence of major bleeding episodes was not significantly increased in the patients treated with aspirin.

Phlebotomy remains the cornerstone of therapy of PV, but additional cytoreductive treatments are required in most patients. Choices of *myelosuppressive agents* include hydroxyurea, radiophosphorus, interferon-α, and anagrelide. Hydroxyurea reduces the thrombosis rate and can normalize the platelet count and spleen size. Because of concerns about teratogenicity and leukemogenicity, the use of hydroxyurea should be limited to patients over age 60. Radioactive phosphorus (^{32}P) is taken up by the bone matrix and locally irradiates the bone marrow, suppressing hematopoiesis. However, ^{32}P treatment is associated with an increased risk of late-occurring acute myelogenous leukemia, and so its use is generally restricted to elderly patients with PV. In clinical practice this agent is now rarely used. Anagrelide is an orally active vasodilator that inhibits megakaryocyte maturation and thus decreases the platelet count. In a study of more than 500 patients with thrombocytosis due to a myeloproliferative disorder, anagrelide was found to reduce the platelet count in over 90%, usually within 2 weeks.

Subcutaneous injection of interferon-α suppresses the proliferation of hematopoietic progenitors, controlling blood counts, splenomegaly, and constitutional symptoms in a majority of patients. Problems with the use of interferon-α include flu-like side effects, slow onset of action (over months), depression, and high cost, limiting its practical use to women who desire pregnancy. Interferon-α has been reported to be safe in pregnancy, whereas the other cytoreductive agents are known teratogens.

The present patient continues to be managed with intermittent phlebotomy, hydroxyurea, and low-dose aspirin, more than 10 years following the date of her original diagnosis.

Clinical Pearls

1. Polycythemia vera (PV) is characterized by an elevated red cell mass in the absence of conditions that induce secondary polycythemia.

2. In PV, erythropoietin (EPO) levels are typically low. In contrast, most acquired secondary causes of polycythemia are associated with elevated or high/normal EPO levels.

3. Phlebotomy remains the cornerstone of therapy of PV, but additional cytoreductive treatments are required in most patients. Choices of myelosuppressive agents include hydroxyurea, radiophosphorus, interferon-α, and anagrelide.

REFERENCES

1. Landolfi R, Marchioli R, Kutti J, et al: Efficacy and safety of low-dose aspirin in polycythemia vera. N Engl J Med 350: 114-124, 2004.
2. Pearson TC, Messinezey M, Westwood N, et al: A Polycythemia Vera Update: Diagnosis, Pathobiology and Treatment. Hematology, American Society of Hematology Education Program Book, 2000.

PATIENT 17

A 16-year-old girl with small bowel obstruction and abdominal adenopathy

A 16-year-old girl with a history of irritable bowel syndrome presents to the emergency department with stabbing periumbilical abdominal pain. Over the previous 3 months she has noted weight loss, progressive abdominal fullness, and two to three loose stools per day.

Physical Examination: Blood pressure 105/65 mmHg, pulse 110, temperature 38.4°C. General: thin; in moderate pain. HEENT: anicteric. Lymph nodes: no adenopathy. Cardiovascular: tachycardic, no murmurs. Chest: clear to auscultation. Abdomen: moderate distention, mild periumbilical tenderness, decreased bowel sounds. Extremities: no edema.

Laboratory Findings: WBC 12/μL (80% neutrophils, 16% lymphocytes), hemoglobin 12.1 g/dL, platelets 350,000/μL. Biochemistry profile: normal. Liver function tests: normal. Chest radiograph: normal. Abdominal CT: small bowel obstruction due to abdominal lymphadenopathy.

Course: The patient is taken to the OR and undergoes segmental resection of the obstructed jejunum and a lymph node biopsy. The pathology of the lymph node biopsy reveals diffuse infiltration of the node by large pleomorphic lymphocytes with horseshoe-shaped nuclei. Immunostains show that these cells are positive for CD30, CD25, and CD3, but negative for CD20 and CD15 (see Figures).

Questions: What is the most likely diagnosis? Which additional tests should one order to distinguish different prognostic groups?

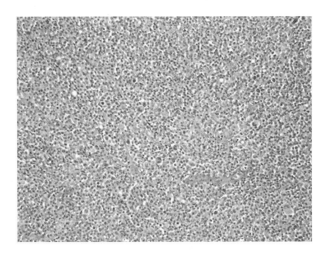

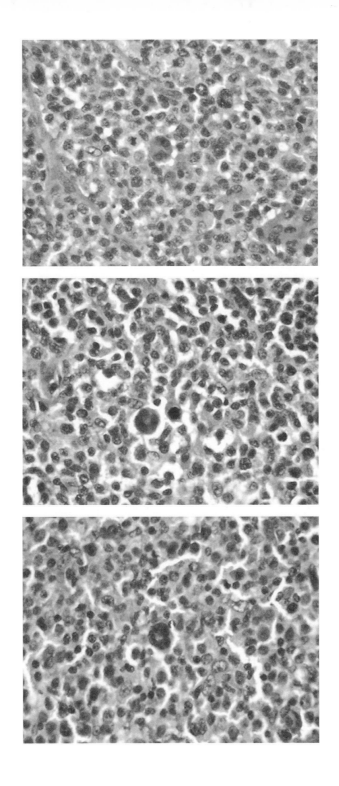

Answers: Primary systemic anaplastic large cell lymphoma, T-cell type, is the most likely diagnosis. Appropriate additional tests to order include CT scan of chest, bone marrow biopsy, and immunohistochemistry to detect the anaplastic lymphoma kinase (ALK) protein.

Discussion: Anaplastic large cell lymphoma (ALCL) of T/null-cell type is a neoplasm of large lymphoid cells expressing CD30 and either T-cell or no lineage-specific antigens involving lymph nodes or extra-nodal sites. ALCL represents approximately 3% of all non-Hodgkin's lymphomas and has a bimodal age distribution. The clinical features of anaplastic large cell lymphoma include frequent involvement of the skin (21%) and other extra-nodal sites, such as the bone (17%), soft tissues (17%), lung (11%), and liver (8%). CNS and GI tract involvement is rare. At the time of diagnosis, most patients have stage III or IV disease. Bone marrow involvement is found in 30% of patients. Constitutional symptoms, particularly fever, are present in about 75% of patients.

In most cases, ALCL is characterized by the chromosomal translocation t(2;5) (p23;q35), which results in a fusion between the anaplastic lymphoma kinase (ALK) gene at chromosome band 2p23 and nucleophosmin (NPM) at chromosome band 5q35. The fusion gene encodes a hybrid protein (p80), in which the amino terminus of NPM is linked to the catalytic domain of ALK, causing constitutive activation of the kinase and phosphorylation of downstream targets involved in malignant transformation.

Morphologically, the tumor is composed of large blasts with pleomorphic, often horseshoe-shaped nuclei with multiple prominent nucleoli. The cells have a moderate amount of mildly basophilic cytoplasm that may contain vacuoles. The hallmark cell of ALCL has an eccentric nucleus and a prominent, perinuclear eosinophilic region. The tumor cells grow in a diffuse, cohesive pattern and commonly infiltrate the lymph node sinuses or perivascular area.

Immunophenotypically, ALCL cells are CD30-positive and express usually CD25 and endothelial monocyte antigen. They are typically CD15-negative. More than 50% express one or more T-cell associated antigen, most commonly the E chain of the T-cell receptor/CD3 complex, but also CD4 or CD8, CD43, and CD45RO. The ALK protein can be detected in approximately 60 to 85% of cases.

The standard treatment regimen used for ALCL is cyclophosphamide, hydroxydoxorubicin, Oncovin, and prednisone (CHOP) chemotherapy, given for six to eight cycles. Treatment results and prognosis are excellent, with significantly better 5-year survival in ALK-positive patients (70-80%) than in ALK-negative patients (33-46%). For this reason, ALK-positive cases are not often included in more aggressive (e.g., upfront transplantation) protocols for T-cell non-Hodgkin's lymphoma.

Additional workup in the present patient included a CT of the chest, which revealed adenopathy in the right perihilar region. A bone marrow biopsy showed no evidence of involvement by the lymphoma. Using immunohistochemistry, the ALK protein was detected in the nucleus and cytoplasm of the anaplastic large cells, and the presence of the NPM-ALK fusion gene was confirmed by reverse transcriptase-polymerase chain reaction.

The present patient was treated with CHOP chemotherapy and achieved a complete remission.

Clinical Pearls

1. Anaplastic large cell lymphoma of T/null-cell type is a rare lymphoma characterized by the expression of CD30 and a T-cell or null phenotype.

2. The typical underlying genetic abnormality is a t(2;5) resulting in the fusion protein NPM-ALK.

3. The presence of the ALK protein is associated with a significantly better prognosis.

REFERENCES

1. Gascoyne RD, Aoun P, Wu D, et al: Prognostic significance of anaplastic lymphoma kinase (ALK) protein expression in adults with anaplastic large cell lymphoma. Blood 93:3913-3921, 1999.
2. Morris SW, Kirstein MN, Valentine MB, et al: Fusion of a kinase gene, ALK, to a nucleolar protein gene, NPM, in non-Hodgkin's lymphoma. Science 263:1281-1284, 1994.

PATIENT 18

A 70-year-old woman with fatigue and splenomegaly

A 70-year-old woman presents to her physician complaining of a 2-month history of progressive fatigue. She also complains of early satiety and discomfort in her left upper abdomen. Her past medical history is significant for hypothyroidism.

Physical Examination: General: no acute distress. Blood pressure 140/70 mmHg, temperature 36.8°C, pulse 70. HEENT: anicteric with no pallor. Lymph nodes: no adenopathy. Cardiac: regular rate and rhythm. Pulmonary: clear to auscultation bilaterally. Abdomen: spleen is grossly enlarged and is palpated to the pelvic brim inferiorly. Extremities: no cyanosis, clubbing, or edema.

Laboratory Findings: Hemoglobin 12.9 g/dL, WBC 3300/μL, ANC 1900/μL, platelets 80,000/μL. BUN normal, creatinine normal. Peripheral blood smear: numerous mature lymphocytes with pale cytoplasm, irregular cytoplasmic borders with villous projections. Flow cytometry: negative staining for CD11c, CD25, CD103, CD5, and cyclin D1. Abdominal CT scan: marked splenomegaly.

Questions: What is the likely diagnosis? What is the treatment for this patient?

Answers: The diagnosis is splenic lymphoma with villous lymphocytes. Splenectomy is the treatment of choice.

Discussion: Splenic marginal zone lymphoma (SMZL) is a distinct B-cell neoplasm that primarily involves the spleen and bone marrow and frequently the peripheral blood. SMZL accounts for 1 to 3% of non-Hodgkin's lymphoma. The median age of patients at presentation is 68 years, with a male to female ratio of 1:1.8.

The clinical hallmark of SMZL is massive splenomegaly. Hepatomegaly can be observed, occasionally, but peripheral lymphadenopathy is extremely rare. Symptoms related to moderate anemia are often reported. Mild neutropenia secondary to splenic sequestration and bone marrow infiltration may be observed. An absolute lymphocytosis is seen in 75% of patients. If villous lymphocytes constitute more than 20% of the lymphoid population in the peripheral blood, the disease is called *splenic lymphoma with villous lymphocytes* (SLVL). Some patients may present with an associated autoimmune condition, such as immune thrombocytopenia or autoimmune hemolytic anemia. Up to 50% of patients are found to have a serum monoclonal component, IgM or IgG, at usually less than 30 g/L.

The bone marrow is invariably involved, and bone marrow biopsy reveals typically an intrasinusoidal infiltration with small lymphocytes. Pathology from splenectomy specimens shows typically a micronodular pattern associated with diffuse invasion of the sinuses. The neoplastic cells occupy both the mantle and marginal zone of the splenic white pulp, with usually a central residual atrophic or hyperplastic germinal center. The red pulp is also involved, with both a diffuse and micronodular pattern and sinus infiltration.

The typical immunophenotype of SMZL is surface IgM-positive, surface IgD-positive, pan B antigens-positive (CD19, CD20, CD22), and BCL2-positive. Lack of CD5 and cyclin D1 allows distinction from mantle cell lymphoma and B-CLL. Similarly, lack of CD103, CD25, and CD11c allows distinction from hairy cell leukemia. In rare cases an atypical phenotype of CD5-positive cells is observed.

SMZL is considered a low-grade lymphoma and has typically an indolent course, frequently requiring no immediate therapy. Five-year survival rates range from 65 to 78%. The indication for treatment is usually the development of cytopenia or symptomatic splenomegaly. When treatment is necessary, splenectomy is the treatment of choice and is considered the best first-line therapy. Sustained improvement in cytopenia and relief of abdominal symptoms are achieved with splenectomy alone in the majority of patients. In patients with medical contraindications to splenectomy, splenic irradiation has been successfully employed.

Chemotherapy involving alkylating agents (cyclophosphamide or chlorambucil) is of marginal benefit. Few patients benefit from these agents when used as first-line therapy; however, in cases of disease progression after splenectomy good partial responses may be achieved with these agents. The use of purine analogs (2-deoxycoformycin and 2-chlorodeoxyadenosine) has also resulted in complete and partial hematological remissions in some reports. Treatment with rituximab and radiolabeled anti-CD20 monoclonal antibodies remains an active area of investigation. French investigators have recently reported that in patients with SLVL and hepatitis C virus infection (HCV), antiviral treatment with interferon-α (with the addition of ribavirin for patients with persistent HCV detected by RT-PCR) results in complete hematological remission in patients achieving a loss of detectable HCV-RNA. Larger therapeutic trials of antiviral therapy in HCV-infected patients with low-grade lymphoma are ongoing.

The present patient was initially treated with 2-CdA. Complete remission was achieved and sustained for 3 years. Upon disease recurrence a splenectomy was performed, and complete remission was achieved for 4 more years. At her most recent recurrence, she was treated with rituximab, cyclophosphamide, vincristine, and prednisone (R-CVP). Complete remission has been sustained for over a year.

Clinical Pearls

1. The clinical hallmark of splenic marginal zone lymphoma (SMZL) is massive splenomegaly.

2. If villous lymphocytes constitute more than 20% of the lymphoid population in the peripheral blood, the disease is called splenic lymphoma with villous lymphocytes (SLVL).

3. SMZL is considered a low-grade lymphoma and has typically an indolent course, frequently requiring no immediate therapy. When treatment is necessary, splenectomy is the treatment of choice.

REFERENCES

1. Franco V, Florena AM, Iannitto E: Splenic marginal zone lymphoma. Blood 101:2464-2472, 2003.
2. Thieblemont C, Felman P, Callet-Bauchu E, et al: Splenic marginal-zone lymphoma: A distinct clinical and pathological entity. Lancet Oncol 4:95-103, 2003.
3. Hermine O, Lefrere F, Bronowicki JP, et al: Regression of splenic lymphoma with villous lymphocytes after treatment of hepatitis C virus infection. N Engl J Med 347:89-94, 2002.

Michaela Liedtke, MD

PATIENT 19

A 42-year-old man with swelling in his neck

A 42-year-old man with no medical history presents with right neck adenopathy. He had first noted a lump approximately 2 months prior while shaving but had not paid any attention to it. His wife, who is a nurse, insisted that he see a doctor. He denies fever, weight loss, night sweats, or pruritus and has not noted any other lymph node abnormalities.

Physical Examination: Blood pressure 125/70 mmHg, pulse 71, temperature 37.1°C. General: athletic physique. HEENT: anicteric. Lymph nodes: right cervical adenopathy involving a single lymph node measuring 2.5 cm. Cardiovascular: regular rate and rhythm, without murmurs. Chest: clear to auscultation. Abdomen: no organomegaly. Extremities: no edema.

Laboratory Findings: WBC 5500/µL (normal differential), hemoglobin 14.5 g/dL, platelets 210,000/µL. Biochemistry profile: normal. Liver function tests: normal. Chest radiograph: unremarkable.

Course: The adenopathy does not resolve after a course of antibiotics, and a subsequently performed excisional lymph node biopsy reveals total nodal effacement by a nodular proliferation of small lymphoid cells. In addition, a few cells (approximately 5%) are characterized by a lobulated and twisted nucleus. Immunophenotypically, these cells are CD15- and CD30-negative and CD20- and CD45-positive (see Figures).

Question: What is the most likely diagnosis?

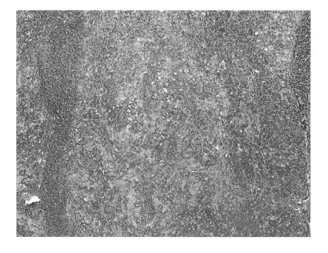

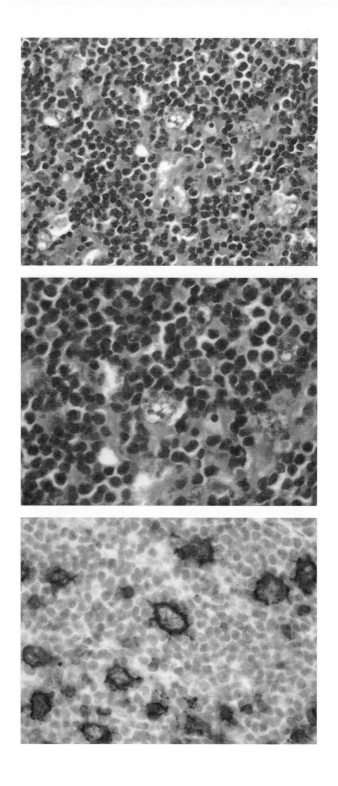

57

Answer: Nodular lymphocyte-predominant Hodgkin's disease is the most likely diagnosis.

Discussion: Nodular lymphocyte-predominant Hodgkin's disease (NLPHD) is a biological entity of B-cell origin that is distinct from classic Hodgkin's disease and its nodular sclerosing, mixed cellularity, lymphocyte-rich and lymphocyte-depleted variants. NLPHD accounts for only approximately 5% of all cases of Hodgkin's disease. It is four times more common in men than in women and reaches a peak age incidence in the 4th decade of life without the bimodal age pattern of classic Hodgkin's disease (HD). At the time of presentation, more than 80% of patients with NLPHD have localized disease, most commonly involving cervical or inguinal lymph nodes and sparing typically the mediastinum. Systemic symptoms and bone marrow involvement are rare.

Morphologically, partial or total nodal effacement by a nodular proliferation of scattered large neoplastic cells in a background of reactive small lymphoid cells is seen. The large cells are called *lymphocytic and/or histiocytic* (L&H) or *popcorn cells* and are characterized by a lobulated and twisted nucleus and a smaller nucleolus than that seen in *Reed-Sternberg cells* of classic HD. The number of L&H cells varies but may reach up to 10% of the cellular population. Classic Reed-Sternberg cells are seen rarely and are not required for the diagnosis. Of note, the small lymphoid cells in the background of NLPHD are polyclonal and are mostly of B-cell origin, thus, allowing a distinction from T-cell–rich B-cell lymphoma, in which the neoplastic B-cells are surrounded by polyclonal T-cells.

In addition to the sometimes only subtle differences in morphological appearance, there are several immunophenotypic and also molecular characteristics distinguishing L&H cells of NLPHD and the Reed-Sternberg cells of classic HD. The typical immunophenotype for NLPHD is CD15-negative, CD20-positive, CD30-negative, and CD45-positive, whereas most cases of classic HD are CD15-positive, CD20-negative, CD30-positive, and CD45-negative. Molecular genetic analysis of single L&H cells have demonstrated somatically hypermutated immunoglobulin heavy chain genes with ongoing somatic mutations within variable (V) region genes, suggesting derivation from centroblasts residing in the germinal center. In contrast, no ongoing somatic mutation of IgV genes is observed in Reed-Sternberg cells of classic HD, consistent with derivation from centrocytes or postgerminal center B-cells.

At the time of diagnosis, patients should undergo a complete staging evaluation, including careful physical examination; CT and PET scans of the chest, abdomen, and pelvis; bone marrow biopsy; and routine blood tests, including complete blood cell count, comprehensive profile, lactate dehydrogenase, and erythrocyte sedimentation rate.

For localized disease, treatment consists of mainly radiation therapy, whereas advanced-stage patients receive combination chemotherapy. Rituximab has recently been shown to have activity in this disease. The prognosis of NLPHD is excellent, and most patients can be cured. Late relapses of NLPHD may occur, but the disease remains generally chemotherapy-sensitive. However, there is a relatively high frequency of secondary non-Hodgkin's lymphoma (3.8% at 25 years), generally diffuse large B-cell lymphoma. The development of secondary non-Hodgkin's lymphoma is usually associated with multiple relapses.

In the present patient, the disease was limited to the right cervical area. He received local radiotherapy and has remained without evidence of recurrence for 2 years.

Clinical Pearls

1. Nodular lymphocyte-predominant Hodgkin's disease (NLPHD) is a rare entity that is morphologically and phenotypically distinct from classic Hodgkin's disease (HD).

2. The disease is characterized by the presence of lymphocytic and/or histiocytic (L&H) cells, also called popcorn cells because of their twisted and lobulated nucleus. Unlike the Reed-Sternberg cells seen in classic HD, the L&H cells are CD15- and CD30-negative.

3. NLPHD is a disease of young people, presents usually with localized adenopathy, and has an excellent prognosis.

REFERENCES

1. Jaffe ES, Harris NL, Stein H, Vardiman JW (eds): WHO Classification of Tumours: Pathology and Genetics of Tumours of Hematopoetic and Lymphoid Tissues. Lyons, France, International Agency for Research on Cancer Press, 2001.
2. Ohno T, Stribley JA, Wu G, et al: Clonality in nodular lymphocyte predominant Hodgkin's disease. N Engl J Med 337:459-465, 1997.
3. Borg-Grech A, Radford JA, Crowther D, et al: A comparative study of the nodular and diffuse variants of lymphocyte predominant Hodgkin's disease. N Engl J Med 318:214-219, 1988.

PATIENT 20

A 68-year-old man with lethargy, clouded thinking, and epistaxis

A 68-year-old man presents with confusion, weakness, and epistaxis of a 3-day duration. Fifteen months ago he underwent a Whipple procedure for localized adenocarcinoma of the pancreas. He developed metastases to the liver and periportal lymph nodes 12 months prior, and he was started on gemcitabine chemotherapy. A partial response was achieved after eight cycles, and because stable disease was evident on his most recent CT scan 1 month prior, gemcitabine was discontinued. He notes decreased urine output but denies any hematuria, melena, rectal bleeding, diarrhea, and easy bruising. Review of systems is otherwise negative in detail.

Physical Examination: General: chronically ill-appearing; no acute distress. Temperature 37.2°C, pulse 85, blood pressure 163/96 mmHg. HEENT: sclera anicteric. Chest: bibasilar crackles. Cardiac: regular rate and rhythm, no murmurs or rubs, no S3 or S4, no jugular venous distention. Abdomen: soft, nontender, no masses or organomegaly. Extremities: trace lower extremity edema bilaterally. Skin: no rash, petechiae, or purpura. Neurological: alert and oriented to person and place only, speech slow, slight asterixis, otherwise nonfocal.

Laboratory Findings: WBC 4500/μL, hemoglobin 7.8 g/dL, MCV 102, platelets 24/μL, BUN 115 mg/dL, creatinine 6.5 mg/dL (baseline Cr 1.5 mg/dL), K 5.3 mEq/L. Total bilirubin 1.6 mg/dL (80% indirect), LDH 553 μ/L, reticulocyte count 5.4%, haptoglobin undetectable. PT/PTT normal. Urinalysis: large protein and blood without casts. Renal ultrasound: no hydronephrosis. Peripheral blood smear: macrocytosis, 2+ schistocytes, 1+ burr cells, and occasional microspherocytes.

Questions: What is the diagnosis? How should the patient be managed?

Answers: The patient has chemotherapy-induced hemolytic-uremic syndrome/thrombotic thrombocytopenic purpura (HUS/TTP), secondary to gemcitabine therapy. Initial management should consist of discontinuation of the offending agent and supportive measures, including hemodialysis, if necessary, to correct electrolyte abnormalities, acidosis, and volume overload. Packed red blood cell transfusions are indicated for significant anemia, but platelet transfusions should be avoided unless necessary for procedures or for life-threatening hemorrhage. Given the patient's fulminant presentation with acute renal failure, severe thrombocytopenia, and mental status changes, a trial of plasma exchange may be warranted. However, although prompt initiation of plasma exchange has become the standard of care for *idiopathic* HUS/TTP, its role in *chemotherapy-induced* HUS/TTP is less well-defined.

Discussion: *HUS* and *TTP* comprise the disorders known as *thrombotic microangiopathies,* which are characterized by abnormal intrarenal and/or systemic platelet aggregation. This leads to thrombocytopenia, intravascular red blood cell destruction, and eventual end-organ damage due to microvascular occlusion by platelet thrombi. Discriminating between TTP and HUS, based on clinical criteria, has been traditionally attempted and widely adopted. However, this distinction remains arbitrary and poorly defined. Because the idiopathic forms of HUS and TTP seen typically in adults demonstrate significant clinical and pathological overlap, they are often considered a single disorder known as HUS/TTP.

The classic TTP pentad of fever, thrombocytopenia, microangiopathic hemolytic anemia, central nervous system abnormalities, and renal failure is actually seen infrequently. It is widely accepted that the combination of a microangiopathic hemolytic anemia (characterized by schistocytosis, reticulocytosis, negative direct Coombs' test, elevated LDH, and decreased haptoglobin) and otherwise unexplained thrombocytopenia is sufficient to make a presumptive diagnosis of HUS/TTP that warrants initiation of therapy. Based on the results of a clinical trial demonstrating higher response rates and survival with plasma exchange compared to just plasma infusion, as well as a decline in mortality rates from 90% to between 10% and 20% since its introduction into practice, plasma exchange therapy has become the standard of care for idiopathic HUS/TTP.

Recently, the underlying pathophysiology behind HUS/TTP has been worked out in some detail. Many patients with both familial and idiopathic TTP have been shown to have a deficiency in a von Willebrand factor-cleaving metalloprotease known as ADAMTS13. This deficiency can be caused by an inherited gene mutation or by autoantibodies against the metalloprotease. Without the metalloprotease, patients are unable to cleave unusually large von Willebrand factor multimers released by endothelial cells and platelets, leading to increased platelet aggregation and pathological microthrombi formation. However, ADAMTS13 deficiency may not be present in "classic" HUS (as opposed to TTP) patients, suggesting that different pathophysiological mechanisms may lead to a similar clinical phenotype, although this awaits further validation in prospective studies.

HUS/TTP due to chemotherapy, as seen in this patient, appears to be a clinical entity distinct from idiopathic HUS/TTP. It should also be distinguished from other forms of drug-induced HUS/TTP, such as quinine- or ticlopidine-associated HUS/TTP, and from cancer-associated HUS/TTP, which is seen occasionally in patients with uncontrolled, disseminated adenocarcinomas and is usually a pre-terminal event. Until recently, the most commonly reported offender was mitomycin C, although cases associated with bleomycin, cisplatin, 5-fluorouracil, estramustine, and interferon-α have also been reported. Although most patients have advanced-stage disease, tumor burden may be minimal, as seen in this case. Features of mitomycin C-associated HUS/TTP include an association with increasing cumulative dose, significant renal failure, and poor response rates to standard therapy, including plasmapheresis, although some success with protein A immunoadsorption columns has been reported. The underlying mechanism of disease induction is poorly understood; direct endothelial damage by the chemotherapeutic agent has been implicated.

Gemcitabine is a pyrimidine nucleoside analog used commonly in the treatment of carcinomas of the pancreas, ovary, breast, and lung. The first case of gemcitabine-related HUS was reported in 1994, and its manufacturer has reported a crude incidence rate between 0.008% and 0.078%. As with mitomycin C, renal impairment is usually a predominant feature, and the incidence appears to be related to cumulative dose/duration of therapy, with a reported median duration of therapy of 7.4 months prior to onset. The onset is typically within a month of the last dose of gemcitabine, although intervals of up to 2 months have been reported. Two distinct clinical courses have been described: an indolent course with gradual development of mild anemia, thrombocytopenia, and renal insufficiency; and a more fulminant course similar to that seen in this case. The former often improves solely with discontinuation of the drug, whereas the latter has a more aggressive course and poorer prognosis.

Treatment for chemotherapy-induced HUS/TTP, particularly for this more fulminant form, is controversial. The experience with plasma exchange in this setting is limited mostly to case series and anecdotes, and, although response rates and survival appear to be poorer than with idiopathic HUS/TTP, significant responses have been reported even in severe cases. Use of protein A immunoadsorption columns in concert with plasmapheresis or exchange has shown some success in small trials, although this technique has not been widely applied. Immunosuppressive agents, such as steroids or azathioprine, have not shown much efficacy in this setting, and novel approaches, such as rituximab, are still being evaluated. Ultimately, the decision to use plasma exchange for chemotherapy-induced HUS/TTP should be made on a case-by-case basis, but for a patient who is rapidly progressing despite aggressive supportive care measures, its consideration is warranted.

The present patient was managed with blood product transfusions and hemodialysis. He did not receive plasma exchange. His platelets recovered over the next 2 weeks; however, he remained dialysis-dependent. He received no further chemotherapy and died 3 months later from progressive pancreatic cancer.

Clinical Pearls

1. Patients with idiopathic hemolytic-uremic syndrome/thrombotic thrombocytopenic purpura (HUS/TTP) present uncommonly with the classic pentad of fever, microangiopathic hemolytic anemia, thrombocytopenia, neurological abnormalities, and renal insufficiency. Having a microangiopathic hemolytic anemia and an otherwise unexplained thrombocytopenia is sufficient for a presumptive diagnosis and initiation of plasma exchange therapy in most settings.

2. Although discriminating between TTP and HUS based on clinical criteria has been widely adopted, significant overlap remains between these two entities. Most clinical presentations consistent with TTP may be due to an inherited or acquired deficiency in the ADAMTS13 von Willebrand factor-cleaving protease. This may not be true for clinical presentations consistent with HUS.

3. Chemotherapy-induced HUS/TTP is a rare but well-described entity, likely distinct from the idiopathic form. Mitomycin C and gemcitabine are the most common inciting agents.

4. Chemotherapy-induced HUS/TTP may have an indolent or fulminant course. Treatment of the former is discontinuation of the chemotherapeutic agent and supportive care, including dialysis, if indicated. Treatment of the latter includes the same plus consideration of plasma exchange in selected patients, although this is controversial.

REFERENCES

1. Moake JL: Thrombotic microangiopathies. N Engl J Med 347:589-600, 2002.
2. Walter RB, Joerger M, Pestalozzi BC: Gemcitabine-associated hemolytic-uremic syndrome. Am J Kidney Dis 40:E16, 2002.
3. George JN: How I treat patients with thrombotic thrombocytopenic purpura-hemolytic uremic syndrome. Blood 96:1223-1229, 2000.
4. Kaplan AA: Therapeutic apheresis for cancer related hemolytic uremic syndrome. Ther Apher 4:201-206, 2000.
5. Fung MC, Storniolo AM, Nguyen B, et al: A review of hemolytic uremic syndrome in patients treated with gemcitabine therapy. Cancer 85:2023-2032, 1999.
6. Furlan M, Robles R, Galbusera M, et al: von Willebrand factor-cleaving protease in thrombotic thrombocytopenic purpura and the hemolytic-uremic syndrome. N Engl J Med 339:1578-1584, 1998.
7. D'Souza RJ, Kwan JT, Hendry BM, et al: Successful outcome of treating hemolytic-uremic syndrome associated with cancer chemotherapy with immunoadsorption. Clin Nephrol 47:58-59, 1997.
8. Rock GA, Shumak KH, Buskard NA, et al: Comparison of plasma exchange with plasma infusion in the treatment of thrombotic thrombocytopenic purpura. N Engl J Med 325:393-397, 1991.
9. Lesesne JB, Rothschild N, Erickson B, et al: Cancer-associated hemolytic-uremic syndrome: Analysis of 85 cases from a national registry. J Clin Oncol 7:781-789, 1989.

PATIENT 21

A 66-year-old man with fatigue and a recent urinary
tract infection

A 66-year-old man presents for evaluation of a persistently elevated white blood cell count. He is admitted to the hospital for a urinary tract infection. He has a several-year history of anemia but has not experienced bleeding or bruising. A bone marrow biopsy 18 months ago was consistent with myelodysplastic syndrome (MDS). The blast count in the bone marrow aspirate was 6%.

Physical Examination: Temperature 36.6°C, blood pressure 146/80 mmHg, pulse 76. General: well appearing, no acute distress. HEENT: mild pallor, anicteric, no adenopathy. Cardiovascular: regular rate and rhythm, without murmurs. Chest: clear to auscultation. Abdomen: nontender, nondistended, no hepatosplenomegaly. Extremities: no cyanosis, clubbing, or edema. Skin: no rashes, purpura, or petechiae.

Laboratory Findings: Hemoglobin 8.9 g/dL, platelets 39,000/μL, WBC 76,200/μL (93% blasts). Biochemistry profile: normal. Liver function tests: normal. Chest radiograph: normal. Bone marrow biopsy: mildly hypercellular marrow with dense infiltration by immature granulocytes, most of them blasts (see Figure). Bone marrow aspirate: 80% blasts; normal cytogenetics. Findings are consistent with acute myeloid leukemia (AML).

Questions: Can the likelihood of leukemic transformation and the median survival be predicted in a patient with myelodysplastic syndrome (MDS)? What are the principles of management of MDS?

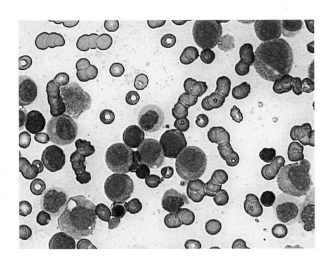

Answers: Yes, the International Prognostic Scoring System stratifies MDS patients into risk categories and allows these predictions. It is a useful guide for disease management. Principles of management include consideration of the patient's age, medical comorbidities, and risk profile in determining therapy, which may include allogeneic stem cell transplantation and/or supportive care.

Discussion: MDS presents with anemia, neutropenia, thrombocytopenia, or a combination of types of cytopenias. The median age of onset is the 7th decade. The basic biology of the disease is impaired cellular maturation in the bone marrow. Such ineffective hematopoiesis results typically in a hypercellular or normocellular appearance on bone marrow biopsy. Various morphological abnormalities in the bone marrow have been described.

Before establishing the diagnosis of MDS, causes of *transient dysplastic changes* in the bone marrow must be ruled out. These include vitamin B_{12} deficiency, folate deficiency, viral infections, chemotherapy, and ethanol, benzene, and lead exposure.

The natural history of MDS can be quite variable, with some patients rapidly progressing to profound cytopenias or AML, while other patients have stable disease for many years. The International Prognostic Scoring System (IPSS), based on analysis of over 800 patients, showed that three major factors determine survival and risk of progression to AML: (a) the percentage of blasts in the bone marrow, (b) the number of deficient hematopoietic lineages in the peripheral blood, and (c) specific cytogenetic abnormalities. This scoring system divides patients into four prognostic risk groups: low, intermediate-1, intermediate-2, and high risk. Patients at low risk have median survival of 5.7 years; high-risk patients have a median survival of 0.4 years.

Disease management should be tailored to the individual patient, taking into consideration the patient's age, medical comorbidities, and risk profile, as determined by the IPSS. Young patients with high-risk disease are candidates for allogeneic stem cell transplantation. Older patients and those with indolent disease may be best managed with supportive care, such as recombinant erythropoietin therapy, packed red blood transfusion, and platelet transfusion, as necessary.

Hypomethylating agents, such as 5-azacitidine, offer a new therapeutic approach for this disease. A recent randomized trial found that time to leukemic transformation or death was 21 months in the 5-azacitidine treatment arm, compared with 13 months in the supportive care control arm.

Once leukemic transformation has occurred, patients can receive standard induction chemotherapy for AML. An anthracycline plus cytarabine is standard induction therapy. Unfortunately, AML arising from MDS is often associated with unfavorable cytogenetics and a lower response rate to chemotherapy than is seen with de novo AML.

The present patient's disease transformed to AML; therefore, he received induction therapy with idarubicin (12 mg/m^2 on day 1) and cytarabine (200 mg/m^2 on days 1–3), followed in 2 months by consolidation with high-dose cytarabine (3000 mg/m^2 every 12 hours on days 1 and 3). Unfortunately, multiple infectious complications developed during consolidation, and supportive care measures were instituted.

Clinical Pearls

1. MDS is characterized by peripheral blood cytopenias and dysplastic changes in the bone marrow.

2. The International Prognostic Scoring System divides patients into four risk groups that predict likelihood of leukemic transformation and overall survival.

3. For young patients, allogeneic stem cell transplant has been the most successful treatment approach. Supportive care is the standard for older patients with indolent disease.

4. Hypomethylating agents are a promising new form of therapy for this disease.

REFERENCES

1. Silverman LR, Demakos EP, Peterson BL, et al: Randomized controlled trial of azacitidine in patients with myelodysplastic syndrome: A study of the cancer and leukemia group B. J Clin Oncol 20:2429-2440, 2002.
2. Heaney ML, Golde DW: Myelodysplasia. N Engl J Med 340:1649-1660, 1999.
3. Greenberg P, Cox C, LeBeau MM, et al: International scoring system for evaluating prognosis in myelodysplastic syndrome. Blood 89:2079-2088, 1997.

PATIENT 22

A 49-year-old man with thrombocytopenia while on prophylactic postoperative low-molecular-weight heparin

A 49-year-old man underwent a mandibular resection for a recurrent head and neck cancer. He received 8 days of postoperative low-molecular-weight heparin (LMWH) as prophylaxis for thromboembolic disease. The patient's platelet count was 317,000 prior to commencement of LMWH. A hematology consult was requested on the 8th day of hospitalization when the surgical team noted that the patient's platelet count had decreased by over 50% to 124,000.

Physical Examination: Vital signs: hemodynamically stable and afebrile. HEENT: anicteric, left mandibular resection site clean. Cardiac: regular rate and rhythm. Chest: clear to auscultation bilaterally. Extremities: trace edema in the lower extremities, no cyanosis.

Laboratory Findings: Hemoglobin 10.8 g/dL, WBC 19, platelets 124,000/μL. PT/PTT/INR: normal. Fibrinogen: normal. Fibrin split products: not elevated. Peripheral blood smear: no schistocytes. Chemistry profile: normal renal and hepatic function. Heparin-dependent antibodies: 2.2 (normal < 0.4).

Question: How should this patient be managed?

Answer: This patient should be managed by stopping LMWH immediately; obtaining a functional or antigenic assay to confirm diagnosis; and addressing anticoagulation issues and selecting a thrombin inhibitor.

Discussion: The diagnosis of heparin-induced thrombocytopenia (HIT) is made clearly based on the temporal relationship of the patient's thrombocytopenia with his LMWH administration and the positive heparin-dependent antibody test. The platelet count associated with HIT begins typically 5 to 10 days after the initiation of heparin therapy. However, some patients will have a more rapid decline and have rapid-onset HIT because of previous heparin exposure. Some patients will have delayed-onset HIT, which manifests itself several weeks after heparin exposure. In HIT, unlike in typical drug-induced thrombocytopenia, the platelet count nadir is typically at 55 to 60 $\times$ 10^9/L. However, some patients may have HIT with a platelet count declining by more than 50% but remaining within normal range. HIT occurs most commonly with unfractionated heparin but may occur with LMWH as well. In addition, surgical patients are more likely to develop HIT than medical patients.

Patients with HIT generate antibodies to the heparin-platelet factor 4 (PF4) complex that leads to formation of immune complexes composed of HIT-IgG-PF4-heparin on the platelet surface that trigger platelet activation. This activation, in turn, results in platelet membrane changes that lead to accelerated thrombin generation. This and other events result in a procoagulant state that is strongly associated with venous and arterial thrombosis (odds ratio 37; 95% CI, 5-1600; $P < 0.001$).

A variety of functional and antigenic assays have been developed for diagnosing HIT. The functional assays measure platelet activation but are technically difficult to perform. These assays include the platelet [^{14}C] serotonin release assay (sensitivity 90-98%, specificity 80-97%) and the heparin-induced platelet aggregation assay (sensitivity 90-98%, specificity 80-97%). The antigenic assays detect antibodies reactive to the PF4-heparin complexes (sensitivity > 90, specificity 50-95%), using PF4 bound to polyvinylsulfonate. A few patients may have clinically suspicious HIT but have a negative antigen assay and a positive functional assay. They may have antibodies to other chemokines, such as interleukin-8 or neutrophil-activation peptide 2.

In patients with isolated HIT (thrombocytopenia alone), approximately 40 to 50% will experience a thrombotic event in the following 3 months, if no therapeutic intervention is undertaken beyond discontinuation of heparin. Therefore, the following approach is recommended: Patients suspected of having HIT should stop heparin immediately. If there *is* otherwise a clear indication for anticoagulation (i.e., patients on heparin or deep venous thrombosis or pulmonary embolism), another form of anticoagulation should be started. If there is otherwise *no* indication for anticoagulation (i.e., patient was transiently on heparin for prophylaxis), no further therapy is indicated until further evaluation is obtained. If after evaluation the diagnosis of HIT is confirmed by laboratory testing, or if the diagnosis of HIT is felt to be highly likely, despite absence of laboratory confirmation, the patient should be anticoagulated for the diagnosis of HIT with an alternative drug.

The two standard drugs used for HIT in the United States are lepirudin (Refludan) and argatroban, both thrombin inhibitors. Lepirudin is a 65 amino-acid molecule that directly inhibits the active site and the fibrinogen binding site of thrombin. The majority of the drug is cleared renally, and the $t_{1/2}$ is lengthened in patients with decreased renal function. The PTT is followed in patients on lepirudin therapy with the goal of a PTT of 1.5 to 2.5 times normal. Patients may develop antibodies to lepirudin. Therefore, the PTT must be followed at least daily on therapy. Argatroban is a synthetic direct thrombin inhibitor (DTI) that reversibly binds to the active site of thrombin. It is excreted through the hepatobiliary route, and the dose should be reduced in patients with hepatic dysfunction. Therefore, argatroban is preferred in patients with renal dysfunction, and lepirudin is preferred in patients with hepatic dysfunction.

Because HIT leads to accelerated thrombin generation, coumadin should not be initiated until the platelet count has recovered because there is a high potential for precipitating a thrombotic event and venous limb gangrene. Patients with HIT should be treated initially with a DTI. After the platelet count has normalized, coumadin may be started with 4 to 5 days of overlap on DTI treatment. Particularly with argatroban, the INR will rise with concurrent argatroban and coumadin treatment. The argatroban can be discontinued when the INR is greater than 4.

The present patient was diagnosed with HIT. LMWH was discontinued. He, subsequently, developed bilateral lower extremity deep vein thromboses and pulmonary emboli and required admission to the ICU for monitoring. He was treated with argatroban and was eventually transitioned to coumadin. He was discharged home on coumadin.

Clinical Pearls

1. Heparin-induced thrombocytopenia (HIT) occurs classically 5 to 10 days after initiation of heparin exposure.

2. HIT should be considered even in patients with a normal platelet count, if the platelet count has decreased by more than 50% from its baseline.

3. In suspected HIT, heparin therapy must be discontinued and anticoagulation begun with an alternative anticoagulant, such as lepirudin or argatroban.

4. Coumadin should not be initiated until the platelet count is normal.

REFERENCES

1. Warkentin TE: Heparin-induced thrombocytopenia and thrombosis. Hematology 2003:503-509, 2003.
2. Warkentin TE: Platelet count monitoring and laboratory testing for heparin-induced thrombocytopenia: Recommendations of the College of American Pathologists. Arch Pathol Lab Med 126:1415-1423, 2002.
3. Greinacher A, Lubenow N: Recombinant hirudin in clinical practice. Circulation 103(10):1479-1484.

PATIENT 23

A 56-year-old man with fatigue, shortness of breath, and jaundice

A 56-year-old man with a history of noninsulin-dependent diabetes mellitus presents to the emergency department complaining of a 1-week history of progressive fatigue and dyspnea on exertion. Over the last 2 days his wife has noticed that yellow sclera has developed. The patient recently completed a course of penicillin for an upper respiratory infection.

Physical Examination: General: ill-appearing. Temperature 37.1°C, blood pressure 130/80 mmHg, pulse 120 regular. HEENT: icteric sclera, pale conjunctiva. Cardiac: tachycardic with grade III/VI systolic murmur. Chest: clear to auscultation bilaterally. Abdomen: soft, nontender, palpable splenomegaly 2 cm below costal margin. Rectal exam: no blood.

Laboratory Findings: Hemoglobin: 6.7 g/dL, platelets 370,000/μL, WBC 11,700/μL. MCV: 130/fl. Peripheral blood smear: numerous spherocytes. Chemistry panel: indirect bilirubin 2.1 mg/dL, reticulocyte count 11%. Direct antiglobulin test: positive.

Questions: What is the most likely diagnosis? What treatment should be initiated for the patient?

Answers: Warm-antibody autoimmune hemolytic anemia is the most likely diagnosis. Glucocorticoid therapy is considered the first-line treatment.

Discussion: Immune hemolytic anemia is caused by antibodies binding the red cell membrane and initiating destruction of red blood cells via complement fixation and/or clearance by the reticuloendothelial system. Autoimmune hemolytic anemia (AIHA) is characterized by self-antibodies directed against specific red cell membrane antigens. These antibodies are typically IgG or IgM. Warm-antibody AIHA is mediated by IgG antibodies, which optimally bind the red cells at 37°C. Cold-reacting antibodies bind red blood cells at temperatures below 37°C and are typically IgM. IgM antibodies are seen with the autoimmune hemolysis associated with mycoplasma infection, Epstein-Barr virus infections, and cold agglutinin disease—a syndrome associated with B-cell lymphoproliferative disorders in elderly patients.

The findings in this patient are in keeping with a warm-antibody AIHA. However, with the recent exposure to penicillin, consideration should be given to the possibility of a drug-induced hemolytic anemia or glucose-6-phosphate dehydrogenase deficiency. Note, however, that these conditions are not associated with a positive direct antiglobulin test; thus, warm-antibody hemolytic anemia is the most likely diagnosis in this patient. Patients with this condition present with symptoms of anemia, jaundice, abdominal pain, and fever. The disorder may be insidious, with a chronic waxing and waning course. Acute presentation with fulminant hemolysis, jaundice, pallor, hemoglobinuria, and splenomegaly may also be seen. Warm-antibody AIHA is usually idiopathic; however, it may be secondary to lymphoproliferative disorders, such as chronic lymphatic leukemia, Hodgkin's disease, and non-Hodgkin's lymphoma.

The anemia may be either normocytic or macrocytic reflecting a reticulocytosis, although reticulocytopenia may be present in patients with intercurrent infection or marrow involvement with neoplastic disease. The blood smear often shows spherocytosis, as demonstrated in the case presented. The comprehensive panel will show an elevated indirect bilirubinemia and elevated LDH. In cases of fulminant hemolysis, haptoglobin is typically reduced, with hemoglobinuria and hemosidenuria seen in the urine. The diagnosis is confirmed by a positive direct antiglobulin test (Coombs' test) in over 95% of cases. The rare cases of negative Coombs' test reflect either very low quantities of IgG autoantibodies or other Ig types, such as IgA and IgM.

The mainstay of treatment for warm-autoimmune hemolysis is with glucocorticoids, such as prednisone. Glucocorticoids interfere with macrophage-mediated clearance of IgG or complement-coated red blood cells. Improvement occurs typically within a few weeks of initiating steroids in 70 to 80% of patients. If the hemolysis persists and remains severe, splenectomy is usually the second-line treatment in patients who are surgical candidates. Splenectomy has a response rate of approximately 75%. Vaccination against encapsulated organisms must occur prior to splenectomy.

Cytotoxic agents are another treatment option for patients who fail glucocorticoid therapy. Cyclophosphamide, azathioprine, and cyclosporine have been used successfully in patients with progressive disease refractory to steroids and splenectomy and in patients who are not surgical candidates. Recently, there have been reports of refractory AIHA responding to the anti-CD20 monoclonal antibody rituximab. Other therapies that have been tried with moderate success include intravenous immunoglobulin, danazol, and vincristine.

In patients with life-threatening anemia, red blood cell transfusions should be given. Panagglutinating warm autoantibodies pose significant difficulties to the blood bank, when attempting to cross-match blood, because the panreactive autoantibody present in the patient's serum can mask an existing alloantibody by making all donor units appear incompatible. To overcome this issue, the autoantibody may be adsorbed from the patient's serum before testing for compatible units, and if transfusion is medically indicated, the "least incompatible" units should be used.

The present patient was treated with a week of intravenous methylprednisolone with little response. His hemoglobin fell as low as 4 g/dL, necessitating red blood cell transfusion. After 2 weeks of steroids, severe hemolysis persisted; he therefore underwent a splenectomy. With a tapering dose of steroids after splenectomy, the patient's hemolysis improved slowly.

Clinical Pearls

1. Warm-antibody autoimmune hemolytic anemia is mediated by IgG antibodies, which optimally bind the red cells at 37°C.

2. The diagnosis is confirmed by a positive direct antiglobulin test (Coombs' test) in over 95% of cases.

3. The mainstay of treatment for warm-autoimmune hemolysis is glucocorticoids.

REFERENCES

1. Gehrs BC, Friedberg RC: Autoimmune hemolytic anemia. Am J Hematol 69:258-271, 2002.
2. Petz LD: Treatment of autoimmune hemolytic anemias. Curr Opin Hematol 8:411-416, 2001.

PATIENT 24

A 73-year-old man with a violaceous nodule on the left temporoparietal scalp

A 73-year-old man noted a new violaceous nodule on his left temporoparietal scalp. After several months, the lesion progressed to approximately 4 cm in diameter. A biopsy was consistent with angiosarcoma of the scalp. A wide excision of the lesion with skin grafting was performed, but the surgical margins were positive. Therefore, external beam radiation therapy (5940 cGy) was administered. Three months after completion of radiation, the patient noticed a new nodule on his scalp within the radiation field. A biopsy demonstrated angiosarcoma. The patient now presents to discuss disease management options.

Physical Examination: General: well-appearing, no acute distress. Vital signs: temperature 36.2°C, blood pressure 110/70 mmHg, pulse 68. HEENT: 3-cm erythematous patch without ulceration in left temporal area; diffuse firmness in left preauricular and left postauricular areas; shotty left supraclavicular lymphadenopathy; anicteric sclerae; oropharynx without lesions. Cardiac: regular rate and rhythm, without murmurs. Chest: clear to auscultation. Abdomen: nontender, nondistended, no hepatosplenomegaly. Extremities: no cyanosis, clubbing, or edema. Skin: no other lesions.

Laboratory Findings: Peripheral blood counts and comprehensive metabolic panel: unremarkable. CT scan of neck: several subcentimeter left posterior auricular subcutaneous nodules; shotty submental, right submandibular, and left supraclavicular lymphadenopathy. Chest X-ray: unremarkable.

Questions: What is the prognosis for the patient? What are the treatment options?

Answers: The overall prognosis for recurrent angiosarcoma is poor, with reported 5-year survival rates of 10 to 35%. If feasible, surgical resection can be considered for localized disease. There is preliminary evidence supporting the use of chemotherapy in this setting, with taxanes as first-line therapy and anthracyclines as second-line therapy.

Discussion: Angiosarcoma is a high-grade sarcoma that arises from vascular or lymphatic endothelium. This is a rare disease, comprising less than 1% of all sarcomas. Angiosarcoma characteristically occurs on the scalp and upper forehead of elderly individuals. Other typical sites are soft tissues, liver, bone, and breast. Most angiosarcomas arise without any known predisposing factors. Rarely, angiosarcoma develops as a sequela of chronic lymphedema or prior radiation therapy. Diagnosis is often delayed due to the variable clinical presentations of this disease. The most important prognostic factor for angiosarcoma is size of the tumor at the time of diagnosis. In a retrospective study of 67 patients by Mark and colleagues, 5-year disease-free survival was 13% for lesions greater than 5 cm and 32% for lesions less than 5 cm.

Surgical resection is the first-line approach for all angiosarcomas. Several cases of long-term survival have been reported for patients who received adjuvant radiation therapy. Chemotherapy is reserved for disease recurrence.

In this case, further radiation therapy would be unlikely to achieve benefit in view of the rapid disease recurrence in a previously irradiated field. The surgical consultant felt that repeat excision would result in unacceptable disfigurement.

There is a limited amount of clinical data on chemotherapy regimens for scalp angiosarcoma. In a single-institution study by Fata and colleagues, paclitaxel resulted in major responses in eight of nine patients. Four partial responses and four complete responses were observed, with median response duration of 5 months (range, 2–13 months). Major responses to liposomal doxorubicin have been described in case reports. Eiling and colleagues found that one patient with radiotherapy-resistant scalp angiosarcoma experienced a complete response after six cycles of liposomal doxorubicin. In a patient with unresectable angiosarcoma of the scalp, Wollina and colleagues noted a stable partial response maintained with 21 cycles of monthly liposomal doxorubicin. The observation that some angiosarcomas express the vascular endothelial growth factor receptor has stimulated interest in the use of anti-angiogenesis drugs for this disease. However, this remains a question for clinical research.

The present patient experienced a near complete response to paclitaxel (175 mg/m^2 every 3 weeks). Response duration was 4.5 months. A second partial response was achieved with doxorubicin (50 mg/m^2 every 3 weeks), with response duration of 11 months. The patient then received paclitaxel again, this time administered as a weekly regimen (90 mg/m^2). Partial response was again achieved, which lasted for 11 months. No responses were seen with subsequent single-agent regimens of ifosfamide and gemcitabine. The patient had extensive local progression of disease, and supportive care was initiated.

Clinical Pearls

1. Initial tumor size at diagnosis is the most important prognostic factor in angiosarcoma.
2. Local control of disease with surgery is the first-line approach.
3. Initial studies suggest that paclitaxel is active against scalp angiosarcoma. Anthracycline-based chemotherapy, such as doxorubicin or liposomal doxorubicin, can be considered as second-line chemotherapy after taxanes.

REFERENCES

1. Eiling S, Lischner S, Busch JO, et al: Complete remission of radio-resistant angiosarcoma of scalp by systemic treatment with liposomal doxorubicin. Br J Dermatol 147:150-153, 2002.
2. Weiss SW, Goldblum JR: Malignant vascular tumors. In Enzinger, Weiss (eds): Soft Tissue Tumors, 4th ed. St. Louis, Mosby, 2001, pp 917-954.
3. Wollina U, Fuller J, Graefe T, et al: Angiosarcoma of the scalp: Treatment with liposomal doxorubicin and radiotherapy. J Cancer Res Clin Oncol 127:396-399, 2001.
4. Fata F, O'Reilly E, Ilson D, et al: Paclitaxel in the treatment of patients with angiosarcoma of the scalp or face. Cancer 86:2034-2037, 1999.
5. Brown LF, Tognazzi K, Dvorak HF, Harrist TJ: Strong expression of kinase insert domain-containing receptor, a vascular permeability factor/vascular endothelial growth factor receptor in AIDS-associated Kaposi's sarcoma and cutaneous angiosarcoma. Am J Pathol 148:1065-1074, 1996.
6. Mark RJ, Poen JC, Tran LM, et al: Angiosarcoma: A report of 67 patients and a review of the literature. Cancer 77:2400-2406, 1996.
7. Hashimoto M, Ohsawa M, Ohnishi A, et al: Expression of vascular endothelial growth factor and its receptor mRNA in angiosarcoma. Lab Invest 73:859-863, 1995.

PATIENT 25

A 32-year-old man with bruising and progressive epistaxis

A 32-year-old man presented to a local emergency department complaining of a 2-week history of easy bruising and worsening epistaxis. Over the preceding 3 weeks he had lost 20 pounds, and he describes drenching night sweats and fevers.

Physical Examination: Temperature 39.7°C, pulse 120, blood pressure 150/80 mmHg. HEENT: anicteric. Nodes: no peripheral adenopathy. Abdomen: soft nontender, palpable spleen tip. Chest: clear. Skin: diffuse ecchymosis.

Laboratory Findings: Hemoglobin 12.1 g/dL, platelets 31,000/μL, WBC 67,000/μL. Biochemistry profile: normal. D-dimer: greater than 20. Fibrinogen 117, fibrinogen split products 160 (elevated). Peripheral blood smear: marked thrombocytopenia and numerous immature-appearing myeloid cells. Bone marrow aspirate: immature-appearing myeloid cells with cleaved and folded nuclei (see Figure).

Questions: What is the most likely diagnosis? What additional studies are required to confirm the diagnosis?

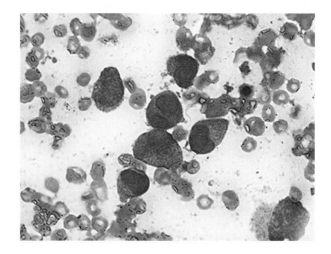

Diagnosis: Acute promyelocytic leukemia is the most likely diagnosis. Cytogenetic analysis to confirm the t(15;17) translocation is required.

Discussion: The French-American-British (FAB) classification divides acute myelocytic leukemia (AML) into eight subtypes (M0–M7), with acute promyelocytic leukemia (APL) as M3 in this classification. APL makes up approximately 15% of AML in adults. The median age at presentation is 40 years, which is much younger than other subtypes of AML presenting typically at a median age of 70 years.

More than 98% of cases of APL have the cytogenetic characteristic of a balanced reciprocal translocation, t(15;17), resulting in the *fusion* of the *retinoic acid receptor-α gene* (RAR-α) with the *promyelocytic leukemia gene* (PML). As a result of this fusion, there is increased affinity of a nuclear corepressor protein complex. This complex attracts histone deacetylase, which further alters chromatin confirmation, leading to the inhibition of transcription and subsequent differentiation arrest. The mechanism of action of retinoic acid in APL is to induce release of the nuclear corepressor complex with histone deacetylase, leading to normal chromatin confirmation, transcription, and differentiation. In a small percentage of cases, the t(15;17) translocation is not detected by conventional cytogenetic analysis or fluorescence *in situ* hybridization (FISH); however, molecular analysis with polymerase chain reaction (PCR) can detect the fusion transcript. Very rare patients are found to have different translocations, resulting in alternative fusion partners with RAR-α. An example of such a variant translocation is t(11;17), which fuses RAR-α with the promyelocytic leukemia zinc finger gene. Bone marrow morphology is characterized by numerous promyelocytes with heavily granulated cytoplasm and cleaved, bilobed, folded nuclei. A microgranular variant exists (M3V), in which the granules are below the resolution of light microscopy.

The clinical presentation of APL is similar to that of other acute myeloid leukemias, with symptoms and signs of bone marrow failure. A unique feature to APL, however, is the high incidence of *coagulopathy* at presentation, leading to a *bleeding diathesis*. Prior to the introduction of all-*trans* retinoic acid, hemorrhagic complications were a major cause of mortality in patients with APL.

The current recommendations for treatment of newly diagnosed patients with APL is induction of remission with *all-trans retinoic acid* (ATRA) and an *anthracycline* (idarubicin or daunorubicin). Several randomized prospective trials have helped define the role of ATRA in induction for APL, demonstrating improved disease-free survival with the combination of ATRA and concurrent anthracycline. Following induction into a complete remission, it is necessary to give postremission therapy with two to three cycles of anthracycline chemotherapy. The goal of such consolidation therapy is the complete eradication of the leukemic clone. Achievement of a molecular remission, as determined by PCR, predicts the likelihood of disease-free survival.

Prospective randomized trials have also demonstrated that maintenance therapy with ATRA decreases the rate of relapse. Combination maintenance therapy with ATRA, 6-mercaptopurine, and methotrexate for 2 years has resulted in the lowest relapse rates.

The major toxicity of ATRA is the *retinoic acid syndrome*, characterized by pleural and pericardial effusions, weight gain, edema, dyspnea, fever, and pulmonary infiltrates. The incidence of this syndrome among patients receiving ATRA induction alone approaches 25%. Concurrent administration of chemotherapy with ATRA is thought to decrease the incidence of the syndrome. The syndrome is effectively treated with dexamethasone, 10 mg twice a day for 3 to 5 days. The routine use of prophylactic steroids to decrease the incidence of retinoic acid syndrome has been employed by some but is not universally accepted as standard practice.

In a patient with relapsed or refractory disease, researchers have reported that *arsenic trioxide* can induce a remission in up to 85% of patients. Arsenic trioxide leads to the degradation of the PML/RAR-α fusion protein, allowing differentiation of the leukemic promyelocyte. This agent also induces apoptosis by the activation of caspases. At present, arsenic trioxide is the treatment of choice for patients with relapsed or refractory disease.

The present patient received induction therapy with ATRA and idarubicin, achieving a complete remission. His course was complicated by severe diffuse intravascular coagulation and a splenic infarction. Because his white cell count was greater than 10,000/μL on admission, he is at higher risk of relapse. He was enrolled in a clinical protocol, investigating the role of the addition of arsenic trioxide and a radiolabeled anti CD33 monoclonal antibody (HUM-195) to standard idarubicin consolidation. He remains in molecular remission 10 months following induction.

Clinical Pearls

1. Most cases of acute promyelocytic leukemia (APL) have the cytogenetic characteristic of a balanced reciprocal translocation, t(15;17), resulting in the fusion of the retinoic acid receptor-α gene (RAR-α), with the promyelocytic leukemia gene (PML).

2. A unique feature to APL is the high incidence of coagulopathy at presentation, leading to a bleeding diathesis.

3. All-*trans* retinoic acid (ATRA) plus idarubicin for induction and anthracycline consolidation, followed by maintenance with ATRA, offer the best disease-free survival in patients with APL.

4. Arsenic trioxide can induce a remission in up to 85% of patients with relapsed or refractory disease.

REFERENCES

1. Lowenberg B, Griffin JD, Tallman MS: Acute myeloid leukemia and acute promyelocytic leukemia. Hematology (Am Soc Hematol Educ Program), 2003, pp 82-101.
2. Soignet SL, Maslak P, Wang ZG, et al: Complete remission after treatment of acute promyelocytic leukemia with arsenic trioxide. N Engl J Med 339(19):1341-1348, 1998.

PATIENT 26

A 64-year-old man with a prolonged activated partial thromboplastin time, undergoing elective total hip arthroplasty

A 64-year-old man is scheduled to have an elective hip replacement operation. His past medical history is significant for mild hypertension only, for which he takes a calcium channel blocker. Surgical history includes appendectomy and tonsillectomy in childhood. Postoperative bleeding complicated neither of these procedures. He denies any history of rectal bleeding, hematemesis, easy bruising, hematuria, gum bleeding, or epistaxis. He gives no family history of bleeding disorders.

Physical Examination: Temperature 36.5°C, pulse 70, blood pressure 140/85 mmHg. General: well-appearing and tanned. HEENT: no pallor or icterus. Cardiac: regular rate and rhythm, without murmurs. Chest: clear. Abdomen: nontender, no palpable organs. Extremities: decreased range of motion in right hip. Skin: no ecchymosis.

Laboratory Findings: Hemoglobin 13.5 g/dL, WBC 9000/μL, platelets 256,000/μL. Prothrombin time: normal. Partial thromboplastin time: 130s. Partial thromboplastin time after 1:1 mixing study: 32. Biochemistry and liver function tests: normal.

Question: What is the most likely diagnosis?

Answer: Factor XII deficiency is the most likely diagnosis.

Discussion: Factor XII (FXII) deficiency is a rare disorder, characterized by a prolonged aPTT that corrects after a mixing study and is not associated with an increased bleeding risk. It was first described in a patient named John Hageman by Ratnoff and colleagues in 1955.

The disorder is generally inherited as an autosomal recessive trait and has been identified in up to 3% of healthy blood donors. It is usually not associated with hemorrhagic manifestations, and there have been no reports of excessive bleeding, even with major surgical procedures. Indeed, it was originally thought that factor XII deficiency might actually predispose to thrombosis. There are case reports of the deficiency occurring in patients with ischemic strokes and other thrombotic events, including acute coronary stent thrombosis. The original patient, Mr Hageman, died from a pulmonary embolism. The mechanism of the increased thrombotic risk was postulated to be deficient fibrinolysis. However, recent surveys of patients with factor XII deficiency have not revealed an excessive rate of thrombosis. Thus, at present, factor XII deficiency is not thought to constitute a thrombotic condition.

Laboratory features are typically a prolonged aPTT that corrects upon mixing with normal plasma. In the case presented, the normal platelet count effectively excludes the diagnosis of diffuse intravascular coagulation. The correction of the aPTT with the mixing study excludes an acquired factor inhibitor, such as factor VIII inhibitor or a lupus anticoagulant. These studies are performed by mixing the patient's serum with an equal volume of pooled plasma from normal donors. Normal plasma contains at least 60% of all clotting factors, and the 1:1 mix results in sufficient clotting factor to produce a normal clotting time. Had an inhibitor been present in the patient's serum, it would exert its effect on the mixture, and the clotting time would not correct.

Factor VIII, IX, and XI deficiencies also present with a prolonged aPTT. However, these conditions are typically associated with a history of excessive bleeding, which is not the case in the patient. A specific FXII assay is required typically to confirm the diagnosis. Normal FXII levels range from 30 to 225 µ/dL. The mean level of FXII in plasma of carriers is 50% of normal. Plasma levels may be as low as less than 3% in severe deficiency. Factor assay is required to differentiate FXII deficiency from prekallikrein and high-molecular-weight kininogen deficiencies, which also present with a prolonged aPTT in asymptomatic patients.

Because the patient gives no history of abnormal bleeding, and there are no significant bleeding complications associated with FXII deficiency, hip surgery may be performed safely in the patient. There is no need to expose him to the infectious risks associated with transfusion of fresh frozen plasma (FFP). Some physicians, however, would transfuse FFP, if factor assay demonstrated a severe FXII deficiency with levels of less than 3% of normal. The present patient had a successful hip replacement surgery with no bleeding complications. He received perioperative FFP.

Clinical Pearls

1. Factor XII deficiency is a rare disorder, characterized by a prolonged aPTT that corrects after a mixing study and is not associated with an increased bleeding risk.

2. The disorder is inherited generally as an autosomal recessive trait and has been identified in up to 3% of healthy blood donors.

3. Factor VIII, IX, and XI deficiencies also present with a prolonged aPTT; however, these conditions are associated typically with a history of excessive bleeding.

REFERENCES

1. Hoffman R, Benz EJ, Shattil A, et al: Factor XI and other clotting factor deficiencies. Hematology Basic Principles and Practice, 2nd ed, 110:1691-1703.
2. Ratnoff O, Colopy JE: A familial hemorrhagic trait associated with a deficiency of a clot-promoting fraction of plasma. J Clin Invest 34:602, 1955.

Jeffrey Halaas, MD, PhD

PATIENT 27

A 68-year-old man with a painless testicular mass

A 68-year-old man palpated a painless left testicular mass. He was referred to a urologist and underwent a left transinguinal orchiectomy. Pathological review showed diffuse involvement with large oval-shaped cells containing open nuclei with prominent nucleoli. The specimen stained positive for CD20, consistent with diffuse large B-cell lymphoma (DLBCL). The patient reported no night sweats, fevers, or weight loss.

Physical Examination: Temperature 37°C, pulse 70, blood pressure 130/80 mmHg. HEENT: anicteric, Waldeyer's ring without mass. Lymph nodes: no palpable peripheral lymphadenopathy. Chest: clear. Cardiac: regular rate and rhythm, no murmur. Abdomen: no masses, no hepatosplenomegaly. Extremities: no edema. CNS: nonfocal.

Laboratory Findings: WBC 8500/µL, hemoglobin 13 g/dL, platelets 423,000/µL, Creatine 1.2 mg/dL, LDH 193 mg/dL. CT scan of chest, abdomen, and pelvis: enlarged retroperitoneal, pelvic, and inguinal lymphadenopathy (no bulky sites). PET scan: extensive uptake in pelvic and inguinal lymph nodes (see Figure). Bone marrow evaluation: no evidence of lymphoma.

Question: What is the proper management of this patient with stage IIEA primary testicular diffuse large B-cell lymphoma?

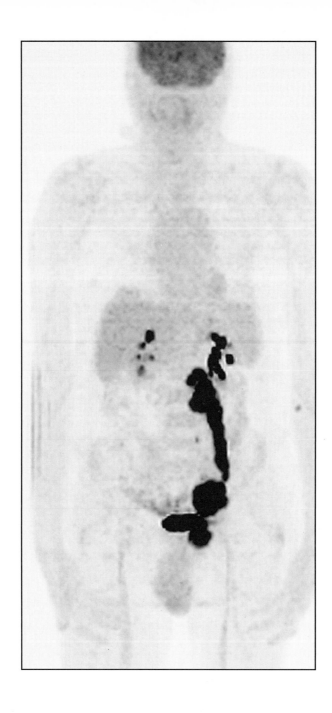

Answer: Following orchiectomy, the patient should receive six cycles of cyclophosphamide, doxorubicin, vincristine, and prednisone (CHOP) with rituximab. Patients with primary testicular lymphoma, who achieve complete remission with anthracycline-based chemotherapy, are at high risk for relapse in both the contralateral testis and the central nervous system (CNS). These represent sanctuary sites protected by the blood-brain and blood-testis barriers; none of the drugs in CHOP are able to penetrate these sites. To prevent relapse at these sites, all patients achieving a complete remission should receive radiation therapy to the contralateral testis and intrathecal prophylaxis with either methotrexate or cytarabine.

Discussion: Primary testicular lymphoma is a rare disease accounting for 1 to 2% of cases of non-Hodgkin's lymphoma. This is a disease of elderly men, with a median age of 66, and is the most common testicular malignancy in men over age 60. Most lymphomas involving the testis are classified as diffuse large cell lymphoma by the WHO/REAL classification system, with other subtypes accounting for 8 to 25% of cases. Testicular diffuse large B-cell lymphoma presents as either stage I or II disease in 55 to 79% of patients. Patients with more advanced stages frequently have involvement of extra nodal sites, such as skin, lung, Waldeyer's ring, and the contralateral testis, as well as the CNS. These latter two sites are often sites of relapse for patients who present with either localized or advanced-stage disease and are important to consider when formulating a treatment strategy for all patients.

Most cases of testicular lymphoma present as a painless mass and are diagnosed by transinguinal orchiectomy. Staging should include CT of the chest, abdomen, and pelvis, as well as bone marrow biopsy and lumbar puncture. Given the rarity of this tumor, there are no published randomized trials to guide treatment decisions, and all the data available are from retrospective reviews. A recent large, international retrospective review by the International Extranodal Lymphoma Study Group (IELSG) has clarified some areas of controversy. In older series, patients with localized stage I or II disease were treated with adjuvant radiation therapy to the retroperitoneum without chemotherapy. However, the high rate of relapse with this approach has led to the use of anthracycline-containing combination chemotherapy in patients with both early- and advanced-stage disease. Although some early, small retrospective reviews gave conflicting results, the IELSG study shows a significant advantage in progression-free survival and overall survival for six or more cycles of anthracycline-based chemotherapy in patients with stage I or II disease, as well as stage III or IV disease. Chemotherapy improves 10-year survival from 19 to 44% for all patients. Treatment of patients with early-stage nodal DLBCL is often with combined modality therapy with short-course chemotherapy (three to four cycles) followed by involved field radiation. However, a retrospective review of this approach showed a higher rate of relapse for primary testicular lymphoma (56%) over other nodal and extra nodal lymphomas (16%), arguing for more extended chemotherapy in patients with primary testicular lymphoma. The addition of rituximab has been shown in the elderly to improve survival in patients with advanced-stage DLBCL. Therefore, six or more cycles of anthracycline-based chemotherapy with rituximab (i.e., R-CHOP) for both early- and advanced-stage disease are considered the standard of care.

Patients achieving a complete remission to chemotherapy remain at risk for relapse, particularly in extra nodal sites. The contralateral testis is often a site of relapse and occurs in 5 to 35% of patients in older series. Furthermore, patients not receiving prophylactic testicular radiation are at continuous risk of relapse, with the risk of relapse reported by the IELSG to be 15% at 3 years and 42% at 15 years. Prophylactic radiation to the contralateral testis reduces the risk of relapse and improves both 5-year progression-free survival (36% vs 70%) and overall survival (38% vs 66%). Therefore, all patients achieving a complete remission with chemotherapy should receive radiation therapy to the contralateral testis. Although radiation therapy to the retroperitoneal lymph nodes has been reported in older series of patients who did not receive chemotherapy, the benefit of adjuvant radiation to these nodal sites is unknown in patients who have received an adequate course of chemotherapy.

The CNS also represents a sanctuary site at significant risk for relapse in patients with testicular diffuse large B-cell lymphoma. The risk of relapse has been estimated at around 10% for early-stage patients and 30% for late-stage patients. In those series characterizing the type of CNS relapse, parenchymal relapse is more common than leptomeningeal relapse. Nonetheless, prophylactic intrathecal chemotherapy is considered the standard of care for patients with primary testicular lymphoma; however, retrospective reviews have been too small to demonstrate a benefit. In the IELSG study, CNS prophylaxis reduced progression-free survival but did not have a statistically significant effect on the risk of CNS relapse or overall survival. This is likely related to the fact that 64% of the patients developing CNS disease relapsed in the parenchyma.

In summary, patients with primary testicular lymphoma of all stages should receive at least six cycles of R-CHOP chemotherapy with intrathecal prophylaxis. Those patients achieving complete remission should by treated with prophylactic radiation to the contralateral testis.

The present patient received six cycles of R-CHOP chemotherapy as well as intrathecal methotrexate. He achieved a complete remission and received prophylactic scrotal irradiation to the contralateral testis. Unfortunately, he relapsed at an extra nodal site in the subcutaneous region of the right thigh. He is presently receiving his third cycle of R-ICE chemotherapy for relapsed disease and will go on to receive high-dose chemotherapy with autologous stem cell support.

Clinical Pearls

1. The most common cause of a testicular mass in men over age 60 is diffuse large B-cell lymphoma (DLBCL).

2. Patients with primary testicular DLBCL have a worse prognosis than similarly staged nodal DLBCL.

3. Patients with early-stage or advanced-stage primary testicular DLBCL should be treated with six cycles of R-CHOP.

4. Patients achieving complete remission from chemotherapy are at high risk for relapse at extra nodal sites and should receive radiation therapy to the contralateral testis and intrathecal prophylaxis.

REFERENCES

1. Zucca E, Conconi A, Mughal TI, et al: Patterns of outcome and prognostic factors in primary large-cell lymphoma of the testis in a survey by the International Extranodal Lymphoma Study Group. J Clin Oncol 21(1):20-27, 2003.
2. Coiffier B, Lepage E, Briere J, et al: CHOP chemotherapy plus rituximab compared with CHOP alone in elderly patients with diffuse large-B-cell lymphoma. N Engl J Med 346(4):235-242, 2002.
3. Lagrange JL, Ramaioli A, Theodore CH, et al: Non-Hodgkin's lymphoma of the testis: A retrospective study of 84 patients treated in the French anticancer centres. Ann Oncol 12(9):1313-1319, 2001.
4. Fonseca R, Habermann TM, Colgan JP, et al: Testicular lymphoma is associated with a high incidence of extranodal recurrence. Cancer 88(1):154-161, 2000.
5. Pectasides D, Economopoulos T, Kouvatseas G, et al: Anthracycline-based chemotherapy of primary non-Hodgkin's lymphoma of the testis: The Hellenic cooperative oncology group experience. Oncology 58(4):286-292, 2000.
6. Tondini C, Ferreri AJ, Siracusano L, et al: Diffuse large-cell lymphoma of the testis. J Clin Oncol 17(9):2854-2858, 1999.
7. Miller TP, Dahlberg S, Cassady JR, et al: Chemotherapy alone compared with chemotherapy plus radiotherapy for localized intermediate- and high-grade non-Hodgkin's lymphoma. N Engl J Med 339(1):21-26, 1998.
8. Zucca E, Roggero E, Bertoni F, Cavalli F: Primary extranodal non-Hodgkin's lymphomas. Part 1: Gastrointestinal, cutaneous and genitourinary lymphomas. Ann Oncol 8(8):727-737, 1997.
9. Moller MB, d'Amore F, Christensen BE: Testicular lymphoma: A population-based study of incidence, clinicopathological correlations and prognosis. The Danish Lymphoma Study Group, LYFO. Eur J Cancer 30A(12):1760-1764, 1994.

PATIENT 28

A 56-year-old woman with an elevated platelet count

A 56-year-old woman with a past medical history of hypertension was noted to have an elevated platelet count on a CBC obtained during a routine evaluation by her internist. She is presently asymptomatic with a negative review of symptoms.

Physical Examination: General: well-appearing, well-nourished. Vital signs: stable. HEENT: anicteric with no pallor. Lymph nodes: no palpable adenopathy. Abdomen: soft, nontender, with no palpable hepatosplenomegaly. Extremities: no clubbing, cyanosis, or edema.

Laboratory Findings: Hemoglobin 12.5 g/dL, WBC 13,800/µL, platelets 1,600,000/µL. Blood film: giant platelets with mild eosinophilia. Iron studies: normal ferritin, normal iron saturation. Bone marrow aspirate: hypercellular marrow with increased numbers of large megakaryocytes; stainable iron present.

Questions: What is the likely diagnosis? What additional tests should be requested? Should this patient's condition be treated now?

Answers: The most likely diagnosis is essential thrombocythemia; however, marrow cytogenetics is required to exclude a diagnosis of chronic myelocytic leukemia (CML) or myelodysplasia. This patient should receive treatment with aspirin and anagrelide or hydroxyurea because she is at risk for thrombotic or hemorrhagic complications.

Discussion: Essential thrombocythemia (ET) is the most common chronic myeloproliferative disorder in the United States, with an incidence of 2.5/100,000. The median age at diagnosis is 60, and the disease is slightly more common in women than men. In one-third of cases, ET is demonstrated to be a clonal hematopoietic condition. Clonality has been associated with an increased risk of thrombotic complications in patients with ET.

At diagnosis, half the patients with ET are asymptomatic, with an elevated platelet count being the only manifestation of the disease. Splenomegaly is present in 25 to 40% of patients. Vasomotor symptoms, such as vascular headaches, visual disturbance, erythromelalgia (burning dysesthesias of hands and feet), acrocyanosis, and seizure may occur with progression of the disease. At diagnosis, up to 25% of patients have had a thrombotic episode. Hemorrhage in the form of GI or oral mucosal bleeding is reported in approximately 5% of individuals, occurring typically when the platelet count exceeds 1,500,000/μL. Women of child-bearing age are at increased risk of first trimester abortions.

To diagnose ET, patients must have a sustained elevation of platelet count above 600,000/μL with no evidence of a secondary cause of thrombocythemia, such as infection, inflammation, recent surgery, malignancy, bleeding, or iron deficiency. Other myeloproliferative conditions, such as CML and polycythemia vera, must also be excluded. The leukocyte alkaline phosphatase (LAP) score is typically elevated in ET but is normal in secondary thrombocythemia. The peripheral blood smear demonstrates usually giant platelets with occasional eosinophils and megakaryocyte fragments. Bone marrow evaluation is important for demonstrating adequate iron stores (excluding a diagnosis of significant iron deficiency) and reveals typically hypercellularity, increased numbers of large megakaryocytes clumped together with hyperploidy nuclei. Marrow cytogenetics must be performed to rule out myelodysplastic syndromes, such as 5q- or CML, which would demonstrate the t(9;22) translocation (Philadelphia chromosome).

Patients with ET can expect a near-normal life span. However, thrombotic complications occur in 10 to 40% of patients within a decade after diagnosis. Patients over age 60 and with a prior history of thromboembolic disease are at particularly high risk for recurrent thrombotic episodes or hemorrhagic complications. Patients less than age 60, with no prior thrombotic episodes and a platelet count of less than 1,500,000/μL, are at low risk of developing thrombotic or hemorrhagic complications. Antiplatelet therapy should be offered to all patients at high risk of thrombotic complications.

Platelet-lowering therapy with hydroxyurea (HU), anagrelide, or IFN combined with aspirin use is the mainstay of therapy in ET. A randomized clinical trial of over 100 high-risk patients demonstrated that keeping the platelet count below 600,000/μL with HU significantly reduced the risk of thrombotic events. Anagrelide and IFN are also useful therapies to decrease the platelet count; however, there is no definitive evidence that decreasing the platelet count with these two agents translates to an improvement in thrombotic risk. The main short-term toxicity of HU is impairment of hematopoiesis, leading to neutropenia and anemia. Less frequent side effects include oral and skin ulcers. There is also concern about the leukemogenic potential of HU, with some studies reporting a higher incidence of AML in patients treated with HU. With the risk of secondary malignancy in mind, HU is generally not recommended for use in younger patients.

Anagrelide is also very effective in reducing platelet counts. Unlike HU, there is no reported increased risk of leukemogenesis with anagrelide use. The most serious complications of the drug are cardiac, including palpations, arrhythmia, and congestive heart failure. When using anagrelide, it is important to aim for a platelet count of 400,000/μL or less, because higher platelet counts have been associated with a persistent risk of vascular complications. The results of the recently reported Medical Research Council PT1 trial in Essential Thrombocythemia demonstrate that compared with HU and aspirin, anagrelide and aspirin are associated with an excess rate of arterial thrombosis, major hemorrhage, and myelofibrotic transformation but decreased venous thrombosis, and suggest that HU should remain first-line therapy in patients with ET at high risk for vascular events.

IFN-α is also an effective platelet-lowering agent. The major advantage of this agent is that it is not known to cross the placenta and is not teratogenic, allowing its use in pregnant patients with ET. Side effects are significant, however, with most patients experiencing fever and flu-like symptoms. Myalgia, weight loss, alopecia, and severe depression are other side effects that result in this agent being discontinued in up to a third of patients.

The present patient was successfully managed with aspirin and anagrelide therapy. She has toler- ated 2 years of anagrelide with only minor symptoms of palpitations, and her platelet count has been maintained at or below 400,000/μL for the last 18 months, with no vascular complications.

Clinical Pearls

1. To diagnose essential thrombocythemia (ET), patients must have a sustained elevation of platelet counts above 600,000/μL with no evidence of a secondary cause of thrombocythemia, such as infection, inflammation, recent surgery, malignancy, bleeding, or iron deficiency.

2. Patients over age 60 and with a prior history of thromboembolic disease are at particularly high risk for recurrent thrombotic episodes or hemorrhagic complications.

3. Platelet-lowering therapy with hydroxyurea, anagrelide, or IFN combined with aspirin use is the mainstay of therapy in ET.

REFERENCES

1. Green A, Campbell P, Buck G, et al: The Medical Research Council PT1 Trial in Essential Thrombocythemia. Blood 104(11), 2004.
2. Spivak JL, Barosi G, Tognoni G, et al: Chronic myeloproliferative disorders. American Society of Hematology Education Program Book, 2003.
3. Storen EC, Tefferi A: Long-term use of anagrelide in young patients with essential thrombocythemia. Blood 97:863-866, 2001.
4. Silverstein MN, Tefferi A: Treatment of essential thrombocythemia with anagrelide. Semin Hematol 36:23-25, 1999.
5. Cortelazzo S, Finazzi G, Ruggeri M, et al: Hydroxyurea for patients with essential thrombocythemia and a high risk of thrombosis. N Engl J Med 332:1132-1136, 1995.

PATIENT 29

A 53-year-old man with a prolonged activated partial thromboplastin time, undergoing elective craniotomy

A 53-year-old man with a history of metastatic anal mucosal melanoma is scheduled to have an elective craniotomy for a solitary brain metastases. Surgical history includes appendectomy and tonsillectomy in childhood, both complicated by excessive perioperative bleeding. He also gives a history of significant epistaxis in childhood and prolonged bleeding after dental extraction. His brother also has a history of childhood epistaxis.

Physical Examination: Temperature 36.7°C, pulse 70, blood pressure 120/85 mmHg. General: well-appearing. HEENT: no pallor or icterus. Cardiovascular: regular rate and rhythm, without murmurs. Chest: clear. Abdomen: nontender, no palpable organs. Skin: no ecchymosis.

Laboratory Findings: Hemoglobin 14.5 g/dL, WBC 8000/μL, platelets 220,000/μL. Prothrombin time: normal. Partial thromboplastin time: 110s. Partial thromboplastin time after 1:1 mixing study: 34s. Biochemistry and liver function tests are normal.

Question: What is the most likely diagnosis?

Answer: Factor XI deficiency is the most likely diagnosis.

Discussion: Factor XI deficiency is an uncommon disorder, characterized by a prolonged aPTT that corrects after a mixing study and is associated with an injury-related bleeding diathesis. It was first recognized as an inherited blood clotting defect by Rosenthal and colleagues in 1953. The bleeding disorder is remarkable for the variability in the bleeding tendency in affected individuals.

Factor XI deficiency is inherited as an autosomal recessive trait occurring most often in persons of Ashkenazi Jewish descent, who have a heterozygote frequency of 9% and a homozygote frequency of 0.2%. At present, four point mutations have been described (termed *type 1* to *IV*), with type II and III mutations accounting for the vast majority of cases in Jewish communities. In homozygotes or compound heterozygotes, plasma factor XI levels are typically less than 15% of normal. In heterozygotes, factor XI levels are 25 to 70% of normal.

Most bleeding episodes in patients with major factor deficiency ($\leq 20\%$ normal) are related to surgery or trauma. Surgical procedures involving tissues with high fibrinolytic activity—such as the urinary tract, nasopharynx, and tooth sockets—are associated with excessive bleeding in patients with severe deficiency. Patients with minor deficiencies have little or no bleeding and are usually heterozygotes for the disorder. However, bleeding tendency does not always correlate with the factor XI level.

The aPTT is prolonged in factor XI deficiency but the PT is normal. As in other factor deficiencies, a 50:50 mix with normal serum corrects the aPTT. A specific assay of factor XI activity is necessary to confirm the diagnosis.

The mainstay of therapy for factor XI deficiency is factor replacement and antifibrinolytic agents. For major surgery, or surgery at sites of high fibrinolytic activity, factor replacement is achieved typically by the use of fresh-frozen plasma for 10 to 14 days with an aim to achieve a trough factor XI level at 45% of normal. Adjunctive use of antifibrinolytic agents, such as epsilon-aminocaproic acid and tranexamic acid may be considered, although their use is relatively contraindicated in genitourinary bleeding. For patients undergoing dental extraction, oral tranexamic acid alone is usually effective in controlling bleeding. A factor XI concentrate is available in Europe; however, a number of thromboembolic events have occurred with this product, limiting its use in the United States. In patients that develop alloantibodies to factor XI, there are reports of the successful use of recombinant factor VIIa to control bleeding.

The present patient was found to have factor XI level of 18% of normal. He received perioperative fresh frozen plasma and had a successful craniotomy with no hemorrhagic complications.

Clinical Pearls

1. Factor XI deficiency is an uncommon disorder, characterized by a prolonged aPTT that corrects after a mixing study and is associated with an injury-related bleeding diathesis.

2. Factor XI deficiency is inherited as an autosomal recessive trait occurring most often in persons of Ashkenazi Jewish descent.

3. The mainstay of therapy for factor XI deficiency is factor replacement and antifibrinolytic agents.

REFERENCES
1. Hoffman R, Benz EJ, Shattil A, et al: Factor XI and other clotting factor deficiencies. Hematology Basic Principles and Practice, 2nd ed, 110:1691-1703.
2. O'Connell NM: Factor XI deficiency. Semin Hematol 41(Suppl 1):76-81, 2004.

PATIENT 30

A 28-year-old man with chest pain and a superior
mediastinal mass

A 28-year-old man with no significant past medical history presents with intermittent chest discomfort increasing over the past 2 weeks. He also notes a 15-pound weight loss and night sweats.

Physical Examination: General: no acute distress. Temperature 36.7°C, pulse 76, blood pressure 150/80 mmHg. HEENT: Anicteric, no tonsillar enlargement. Cardiac: regular rate and rhythm, without murmurs. Chest: clear to auscultation. Abdomen: soft, no hepatosplenomegaly. Extremities: no edema. Lymph nodes: no significant lymphadenopathy.

Laboratory Findings: WBC 8200/μL, hemoglobin 13.5 g/dL, platelets 364,000/μL, ESR 66 mm/hr, LDH 366 units/L. Electrolytes and liver function tests normal. EKG: normal sinus rhythm at 72 beats per minute. Chest CT scan: large anterior superior mediastinal mass on the left compressing the left main pulmonary artery (see Figure). Anterior mediastinoscopy (Chamberlain procedure): large lymphocytes, immunohistochemical stains: positive for CD20, LCA, and BCL-6; negative for CD3, CD5, CD15, CD30, ALK, and BCL-2.

Questions: What is the most likely diagnosis? What is the next step in management?

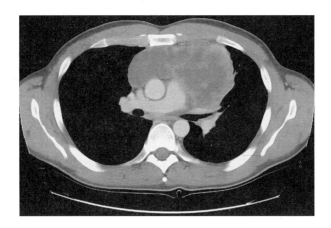

Answers: Primary mediastinal large B-cell lymphoma is the likely diagnosis. The initial treatment recommended for the patient is R-CHOP chemotherapy.

Discussion: Primary mediastinal large B-cell lymphoma (PMLBCL) is a distinct subtype of diffuse large B-cell lymphoma (DLBCL) that makes up 7% of DLBCL and 2% of all non-Hodgkin's lymphomas (NHL). PMLBCL occurs in younger patients (usually in their early 30s), with most series showing female predominance. The anterior mediastinal mass originates in thymus, grows rapidly, and frequently presents with airway compromise and superior vena cava syndrome.

PMLBCL is thought to originate from a thymic B-cell. The lymphoma cells are large, often with clear cytoplasm and surrounding sclerosing stroma that compartmentalizes cells into nests. The cells express B-cell antigens (CD19, CD20, CD22) and CD45 (LCA), but not CD15 or immunoglobulin. Immunoglobulin genes are rearranged. Unlike DLBCL, there are usually no BCL-6 or BCL-2 rearrangements. Gains of chromosome 9p have been described. Recent gene expression profiling studies show that PMLBCL shares features with classic Hodgkin's lymphoma (cHL), such as activation of NF-κB pathway and lower expression levels of B-cell receptor signaling components.

Initial treatment usually includes CHOP with rituximab. Functional imaging such as PET or gallium scans is often used to assess response.

Five-year overall survival in PMLBCL is approximately 50% (similar to DLBCL in general).

Risk factors for relapse include bulky mass, pericardial or pleural effusions, and high International Prognostic Index (IPI) score. Relapses are frequently extranodal. Strategies to reduce relapse include consolidation radiotherapy (especially with bulky disease), more intensive chemotherapeutic regimens, such as MACOP-B, and high-dose chemotherapy with autologous stem cell transplantation (ASCT). In a retrospective review of MD Anderson ASCT data for all DLBCL, PMLBCL predicted better overall survival. A study of 35 patients with PMLBCL transplanted in first remission showed 5 year disease-free survival of 83%.

The present patient had stage IIXBE disease with an increased risk for relapse due to bulky presentation. He was started on an investigational protocol incorporating 4 cycles of accelerated R-CHOP given every 2 weeks with G-CSF support. Restaging PET scan showed mild residual uptake in the mediastinum, but a biopsy revealed only necrosed lymphoma tissue. The patient then received three cycles of ICE. Unfortunately, his follow-up PET scan one month later revealed recurrent uptake in the mediastinum, and a biopsy confirmed refractory disease. The patient underwent autologous stem cell transplantation.

Clinical Pearls

1. Primary mediastinal large B-cell lymphoma (PMLBCL) is a distinct subset representing 7% of all diffuse large B-cell lymphomas and 2% of non-Hodgkin's lymphomas. Gene expression profiling studies show that PMLBCL shares features with classical Hodgkin lymphoma.

2. Patients usually present in their early 30's with a quickly growing anterior mediastinal mass that often lead to superior vena cava syndrome and respiratory compromise.

3. Tumors consist of large cells, often with clear cytoplasm and surrounding sclerosing stroma. Cells stain positive for B-cell antigens (CD19, CD20, CD22), CD45, but not for Ig or CD15.

5. Prognosis and treatment are generally similar to that of diffuse large B-cell lymphoma, with current investigations focusing on more intensive first-line treatment.

REFERENCES

1. Savage KJ, Monti S, Kutok JL, et al: The molecular signature of mediastinal large B-cell lymphoma differs from that of other diffuse large B-cell lymphomas and shares features with classical Hodgkin lymphoma. Blood 102(12):3871-3879, 2003.
2. Van Besien K, Kelta M, Bahaguna P: Primary mediastinal B-cell lymphoma: a review of pathology and management. J Clin Oncol 19(6):1855-1864, 2001.
3. Sehn LH, Antin JH, Shulman LN, et al: Primary diffuse large B-cell lymphoma of the mediastinum: outcome following high-dose chemotherapy and autologous hematopoietic cell transplantation. Blood 91(2):717-723, 1998.
4. Lazzarino M, Orlandi E, Paulli M, et al: Treatment outcome and prognostic factors for primary mediastinal (thymic) B-cell lymphoma: a multicenter study of 106 patients. J Clin Oncol 15(4):1646-1653, 1997.

PATIENT 31

A 46-year-old woman with appendicitis and colonic wall thickening

A 46-year-old woman is experiencing acute severe abdominal pain accompanied by nausea and vomiting. A CT scan reveals an abnormal, thick-walled, enhancing appendix; moderate pelvic free fluid; multiple low attenuation lesions in the liver; and possible wall thickening at the cecal base. She is taken to the operating room the next day for suspected appendicitis.

Physical Examination: General: well-nourished, no acute distress. Temperature 36.9°C, blood pressure 100/60 mmHg, pulse 72, weight 53.7 kg. HEENT: anicteric sclerae, no pallor, no lymphadenopathy. Cardiac: regular rate and rhythm, with no murmurs. Chest: clear to auscultation bilaterally. Abdomen: active bowel sounds with a well-healed small scar around her umbilicus and laparotomy scars in both lower abdominal quadrants; no hepatosplenomegaly or distention. Extremities: no edema.

Laboratory Findings: Electrolytes and transaminases: normal. Pathology: acute appendicitis with focal fat necrosis near the appendiceal orifice; cecal tissue shows infiltrating moderately differentiated adenocarcinoma with a mucinous component comprising less than 50% of tumor. Tumor extends through bowel wall and into pericolic soft tissue. Tumor margins negative. Possible prior perforation at tumor site. Five out of 15 lymph nodes positive. Liver biopsies: evidence of cysts only.

Questions: At which stage is the patient's disease? What treatment (if any) do you recommend now?

Answers: The patient has stage IIIC colon cancer. Adjuvant chemotherapy is recommended.

Discussion: The patient has both acute appendicitis and stage IIIC colon cancer. Her appendicitis was definitively treated with surgical resection. However, such was not the case for her locally advanced neoplasm. The close proximity of her tumor and appendix suggested that the cancer may have caused obstruction of the appendiceal orifice, leading to appendicitis.

Results of a colon pathology examination indicate whether adjuvant chemotherapy is warranted. This patient had several poor prognostic factors that were directly related to the stage of her disease: Tumors extending into the muscularis propria are classified as stage T3, while tumors extending through the muscularis propria and into the pericolic soft tissue are T4 (both are associated with less favorable outcomes). She had five lymph nodes involved with cancer, which, according to the American Joint Committee on Cancer, yields a diagnosis of N2 disease (with four lymph nodes being the cutoff between N1 and N2 disease). In the absence of any metastatic disease, her overall stage was therefore IIIC. The probable perforation was also a poor prognostic factor. Due to her node-positive disease, relative young age, and otherwise good health, adjuvant chemotherapy was warranted.

The current standard of care for patients with stage IIIC disease includes 5-fluorouracil and leucovorin. Studies dating from the 1980s have demonstrated a reproducible survival benefit in patients with node-positive disease. Because these agents do not completely prevent recurrent disease, additional therapies have been evaluated in combination with 5-fluorouracil and leucovorin. For example, oxaliplatin and irinotecan have shown promise in improving progression-free survival and overall survival in patients with stage IV colon cancer, as well as some benefits in earlier-stage disease. In the adjuvant setting, oxaliplatin in combination with fluorouracil and leucovorin has been found to decrease the risk of recurrence in the first 3 years after resection, without clear survival benefits. Data for irinotecan in combination with fluorouracil and leucovorin in the adjuvant setting are still immature.

For this patient, after completing adjuvant chemotherapy, surveillance to monitor for recurrence or a new primary lesion should involve a colonoscopy 1 year after her resection. If the colonoscopy is normal, she will be due for another in 3 years, then every 5 years. Serum CEA levels may be monitored, although this blood test is not used as a diagnostic tool, but rather to follow patients through treatment or to monitor for recurrence. Liver function tests, CT scans of the abdomen and pelvis, and chest X-rays are considered to be less accurate than serum CEA for diagnosing recurrences. Close follow-up with an oncologist is recommended every 3 to 6 months for the first 3 years.

Screening for her family members, assuming that this is a sporadic case of colon cancer, should include full colonoscopies for all first-degree relatives beginning at an age 10 years younger than the age at which this patient was diagnosed. Any additional diagnoses of colon cancer or other types of cancer associated with familial syndromes should prompt consideration for an evaluation of family members by a clinical geneticist.

In the general population, in the absence of a significant family history or personal history of gastrointestinal disorders or malignancy, screening for colon cancer is otherwise recommended to begin at age 50. This screening may occur in the form of yearly fecal occult blood testing (FOBT), flexible sigmoidoscopy every 3 to 5 years, the combination of the two, or colonoscopy every 5 to 10 years.

Clinical Pearls

1. Adjuvant chemotherapy is warranted in patients with resected stage IIIC colon cancer.

2. Regular follow-up with colonoscopy, CEA, and clinical evaluation are warranted in patients with treated stage III colon cancer.

REFERENCES

1. de Gramont A, Banzi M, Navarro M: Oxaliplatin/5-FU/LV in adjuvant colon cancer: Results of the international randomized mosaic trial. Proc Am Soc Clin Oncol 22:253[Abstract 1015], 2003.
2. Wolmark N, Rockette H, Fisher B: The benefit of leucovorin-modulated fluorouracil as postoperative adjuvant therapy for primary colon cancer: Results from national Surgical Adjuvant Breast and Bowel Project protocol C-03. J Clin Oncol 11:1879-1887, 1993.
3. Laurie JA, Moertel CG, Fleming TR: Surgical adjuvant therapy of large-bowel carcinoma: An evaluation of levamisole and the combination of levamisole and fluorouracil. The North Central Cancer Treatment Group and the Mayo Clinic. J Clin Oncol 7:1447-1450, 1989.

PATIENT 32

A 21-year-old woman with constipation and ascites

A 21-year-old woman had been experiencing constipation over a 3-month period. Abdominal bloating then developed, and she presented to an emergency department, where she was found to have ascites. She underwent abdominal paracentesis.

Physical Examination: General: ill-appearing, mild distress. Temperature 36.6°C, blood pressure 120/90 mmHg, pulse 143, weight 74.5 kg. HEENT: anicteric sclerae, mucus membranes dry, no adenopathy. Cardiac: tachycardic, regular rhythm, with no murmurs. Chest: clear to auscultation bilaterally. Abdomen: active bowel sounds, ascites present, no hepatosplenomegaly. Extremities: 2+ bilateral lower extremity edema.

Laboratory Findings: Electrolytes: normal. AST 37, ALT 58, alkaline phosphatase 54, total bilirubin 0.8. Serum carcinoembryonic antigen (CEA) 20. Ascitic fluid: WBC 1580, RBC 2000, 47% lymphocytes, 2% eosinophils, 47% monocytes, 4% mesothelial cells. Ascites fluid cytology positive for adenocarcinoma with signet ring cell features, with positive staining for CEA.

Questions: What is the most likely diagnosis? What additional tests are recommended?

Answers: The patient most likely has metastatic colon cancer, although the differential diagnosis includes other types of adenocarcinoma with signet ring features, such as breast, gastric, and appendiceal cancer. Imaging of the chest, abdomen, and pelvis with CT scan and sigmoidoscopy can assist in confirming the diagnosis.

Discussion: The patient has ascites fluid cytology positive for adenocarcinoma, although there is not sufficient information to determine the tissue of origin. The signet ring cell features are suggestive of colorectal, breast, appendiceal, or gastric cancer (or, more rarely, pancreatic, gallbladder, or ovarian cancer). Her CEA is elevated, consistent with a GI source.

In the evaluation of this patient, a CT scan of the abdomen and pelvis was obtained, revealing a large annular constricting lesion in the distal colon, thickened omentum, and ascites. A flexible sigmoidoscopy revealed a friable thickened mucosal lesion, located 14 cm from the anal canal and nearly obstructing the lumen. A biopsy confirmed adenocarcinoma with signet ring cell features, poorly differentiated. Esophagogastroduodenoscopy was not performed.

Colorectal cancer is the third most common type of cancer in the United States, with approximately 150,000 new cases in 2003. This disease is more common in the elderly and in patients with a family history of colon cancer or such familial disorders as hereditary nonpolyposis colon cancer (HNPCC) or familial adenomatous polyposis (FAP). This patient had no family history of colon cancer. Her symptoms of bowel irregularity are a common symptom of colorectal cancer, albeit not specific.

At diagnosis, stage IV disease had already developed, with metastatic spread to the peritoneum. In patients with such advanced disease, resection is not indicated except for palliative purposes, such as bleeding, perforation, or obstruction. Because of her near-obstructing lesion, this patient did undergo resection with a sigmoid loop colostomy and omentectomy. Once recovered from the operation, systemic treatment with chemotherapy was recommended for her metastatic disease.

The current standard of care for chemotherapy in metastatic colorectal carcinoma includes infusional 5-fluorouracil and leucovorin with either oxaliplatin (FOLFOX regimens), or with irinotecan (FOLFIRI regimen). Data have demonstrated improved progression-free survival, overall survival, and risk reduction for these combinations over the previous standard of 5-fluorouracil and leucovorin alone. Recently, the FDA has approved bevacizumab, a monoclonal antibody against the vascular endothelial growth factor receptor, as an added first-line therapy. As a second-line therapy, the FDA has approved cetuximab, a monoclonal antibody against the epidermal growth factor receptor.

Overall, this patient has several poor prognostic factors, including her advanced stage at presentation, presence of a near-obstructing lesion, elevated preoperative CEA, and histological signet ring cell features. For her, the goals of treatment are palliative in intent, and survival is likely to be measured in the 1- to 2-year range. Screening for her family members should be fairly aggressive because of her young age at diagnosis. The absence of multiple polyps in her colon excludes a diagnosis of adenomatous polyposis syndromes, such as FAP, Gardner's syndrome, and Turcot's syndrome. The absence of cancer in any additional family members makes a diagnosis of the nonpolyposis genetic syndromes less likely. However, all of her first-degree relatives should undergo a screening colonoscopy at an age 10 years younger than her age at diagnosis and receive repeat screening colonoscopies every subsequent 5 to 10 years. If any additional cases of colon cancer are discovered in her family, consideration for a genetic syndrome should be entertained with appropriate referral to a genetic counseling center.

Clinical Pearls

1. Treatment for metastatic colorectal carcinoma includes palliative chemotherapy.
2. Relatives of patients diagnosed with colorectal cancer should undergo screening colonoscopies beginning at an age 10 years younger than the patient's age at diagnosis.

REFERENCES

1. Goldberg RM, Sargent DJ, Morton RF: A randomized controlled trial of fluorouracil plus leucovorin, irinotecan, and oxaliplatin combinations in patients with previously untreated metastatic colorectal cancer. J Clin Oncol 1:23-30, 2004.
2. de Gramont A, Figer A, Seymour M: Leucovorin and fluorouracil with or without oxaliplatin as first-line treatment in advanced colorectal cancer. J Clin Oncol 18:2938-2947, 2000.
3. Douillard JY, Cunningham D, Roth AD: Irinotecan combined with fluorouracil compared with fluorouracil alone as first-line treatment for metastatic colorectal cancer: A multicentre randomized trial. Lancet 355:1041-1047, 2000.

PATIENT 33

A 65-year-old man with increased constipation

A 65-year-old man without any significant medical history presents with 3 months of increased constipation. A colonoscopy shows an obstructing lesion 10 cm from the anal verge. Biopsy of the lesion confirms adenocarcinoma. CT scans of the chest, abdomen, and pelvis demonstrate the presence of a large, 7 cm × 4 cm mass at the rectosigmoid junction as well as one enlarged lymph node, but no evidence of metastatic disease. Surgical evaluation concludes that sphincter-preserving surgery is technically not feasible.

Physical Examination: Temperature 37°C, blood pressure 136/76 mmHg, pulse 84. General: well-appearing, no acute distress. HEENT: mild pallor, anicteric, no adenopathy. Cardiovascular: regular rate and rhythm, without murmurs. Chest: clear to auscultation. Abdomen: nontender, mild distention, no hepatosplenomegaly, no masses appreciated. Rectal exam: no palpable mass. Extremities: no cyanosis, clubbing, or edema. Skin: no rashes, purpura, or petechiae.

Laboratory Findings: Hemoglobin 11.5 g/dL, platelets 252,000/µL, WBC 8200/µL (normal differential). Biochemistry profile: normal. Liver function tests (including LDH): normal. CEA: 8.7 ng/mL (normal 0–5).

Questions: Does this patient have colon cancer or rectal cancer? What is the stage? What is the appropriate treatment?

Answers: The patient most likely has rectal cancer. This is a stage III tumor. Treatment options are surgical resection with preoperative chemoradiation or with postoperative chemoradiation.

Discussion: The site of the lesion, 10 cm from the anal verge, indicates rectal cancer. At presentation, approximately 43% of patients complain of a change in bowel habits, including constipation frequently alternating with diarrhea, and changes in stool caliber. Tenesmus is also a common presenting symptom and is described as a sense of urgency and inadequate emptying of the rectum. Urinary symptoms, buttock pain, and perineal pain are often indicators of more locoregionally advanced disease. Compared to colon cancer, tumors arising in the rectosigmoid area are more likely to present with symptoms. They are also more likely to be associated with rectal bleeding, though less frequently with anemia than right-sided colon cancers. Symptoms at diagnosis generally portend a worse prognosis.

The patient has an elevated CEA of 8.7 ng/mL. Tumor markers have a low diagnostic ability to detect primary colorectal tumors because they can overlap with benign disease and have low sensitivity for early disease. They are not used as screening tests. Serum levels of CEA, however, do have prognostic significance in newly diagnosed rectal cancer. A CEA level greater than 5 ng/mL is associated with a worse prognosis than a normal level for a similarly staged tumor.

In this case, the patient's tumor begins within the middle third of the rectum (approximately 8–12 cm from the anal verge) and extends proximally to involve the recto-sigmoid junction. The rectum measures approximately 15 cm and is divided into thirds for purposes of anatomical localization. The location of the anal verge has significant variation between individuals and is generally not a reproducible landmark. The dentate line, where the squamous mucosa of the anus transitions to the columnar mucosa of the rectum, is a more reliable landmark. Distal cancers within the rectum have a worse prognosis than more proximal lesions.

For further characterization of the tumor stage as either IIIA, B or C, a pathological diagnosis after surgery is necessary. Additionally, a transrectal ultrasound with or without an MRI can be performed to complete clinical staging.

As more patients are considered for preoperative treatment (radiotherapy with or without chemotherapy), clinical assessment has become increasingly important. Preoperative clinical staging includes physical exam, CT scan, and endorectal ultrasound (EUS). The sensitivity of CT for detecting distant metastases is higher than for detecting nodal involvement or the depth of transmural invasion. The sensitivity of CT for detection of malignant lymph nodes is higher for rectal cancers than for colon cancers, and any perirectal adenopathy is presumed to be malignant because benign adenopathy is not usually observed in this area.

EUS is more accurate for staging the depth of transmural invasion (T stage) than CT, though it is similar to CT for detection of perirectal nodal involvement. In one study, the use of EUS affected a change in management in one-third of patients, primarily because CT tended to underestimate the T stage. Recent data suggest that MRI is a more accurate modality for preoperative staging compared to EUS.

Two staging systems (see Tables 1 through 2) are used to assess the extent of disease at presentation: the Duke's classification and the TNM staging system of the American Joint Committee on Cancer. The most recent 2002 version of the TNM system is currently the preferred staging system. In the United States, 34% of rectal cancers are localized to the mucosa or submucosa (Dukes' A or TNM stage I); 25% extend into or through the muscle layer without lymph node involvement (Dukes' B or TNM stage II); 26% have lymph node involvement (Dukes' C or TNM stage III); and 15% have distant metastases (Dukes' D or TNM stage IV).

Five-year survival rates among patients with stage III disease are variable, and the recognition that different subgroups have different prognoses was reflected in the modification of the TNM staging system in 2002, when stage III disease was subdivided into A, B, and C categories. Stage IIIA (T_{1-2}, N_1) had a 5-year survival rate of 55%; stage IIIB (T_{3-4}, N_1), 35.5%; and stage IIIC (any T, N_2), 24.5%. These outcomes were based on studies of patients who underwent surgery without

Table 1. Astler Coller Modification of Dukes' Staging System for Colorectal Cancer

A	Mucosal; above muscularis propria, no involvement of lymph nodes
B_1	Into muscularis propria but above pericolic fat, no involvement of lymph nodes
B_2	Into pericolic or perirectal fat, no involvement of lymph nodes
C_1	Same penetration as B_1 with nodal metastases
C_2	Same penetration as B_2 with nodal metastases
D	Distant metastases

Table 2. TNM Staging System for Colorectal Cancer*

Primary Tumor (T)

T_{is}	Carcinoma in situ; intraepithelial or invasion of lamina propria (intramucosal)
T_1	Tumor invades submucosa
T_2	Tumor invades muscularis propria
T_3	Tumor invades through the muscularis propria into the subserosa, or into nonperitonealized pericolic or perirectal tissues
T_4	Tumor directly invades other organs or structures and/or perforates visceral peritoneum

Regional Lymph Node (N)

N_x	Regional lymph nodes cannot be assessed
N_0	No regional nodal metastases
N_1	Metastasis in 1 to 3 regional lymph nodes
N_2	Metastasis in 4 or more regional lymph nodes

Distant Metastasis (M)

M_x	Distant metastasis cannot be assessed
M_0	No distant metastasis
M_1	Distant metastasis
Stage O	$T_{is} N_0 M_0$
Stage I	$T_{1-2} N_0 M_0$
Stage IIa	$T_3 N_0 M_0$
Stage IIB	$T_4 N_0 M_0$
Stage IIIA	$T_{1-2} N_1 M_0$
Stage IIIB	$T_{3-4} N_1 M_0$
Stage IIIC	Any T $N_2 M_0$
Stage IV	Any T any N M_1

*American Joint Committee on Cancer.

neoadjuvant treatment. It is currently difficult to predict outcomes in patients who undergo pathological staging after preoperative treatment as more data are needed.

It is estimated that 40,500 patients will be diagnosed with rectal cancer in the United States in 2004. Surgical resection is the primary treatment modality for rectal cancer, and outcome is most closely associated with the extent of disease at presentation.

In the present patient, surgeons concluded that sphincter-preserving surgery was not feasible. There are two conventional treatment options for this patient with a clinically resectable rectal cancer. The patient may be a candidate for pre-operative chemoradiation to facilitate a curative resection and to increase the chance of performing sphincter-preserving surgery (by clinically down-staging the tumor). The other conventional option is surgical resection (with abdominal perineal resection) followed by adjuvant therapy with chemoradiation. The decision as to which modality to use often varies according to the institution and surgeon.

Abdominal perineal resection was the gold standard for management of rectal cancer until sphincter preservations were introduced in the early 1950s. Technical advances, including total mesorectal excision (TME) and autonomic nerve preservation, have dramatically decreased local recurrence rate and perioperative morbidity. TME is the standard therapy for mid- and lower-third rectal cancers.

After surgical resection, postoperative chemoradiation has been shown to improve disease control (local and distant), disease-free survival (DFS), and overall survival (OS). Randomized studies from the Gastrointestinal Tumor Study Group, the Mayo/North Central Cancer Treatment Group, and from Norway demonstrated improved OS and local control for patients treated with postoperative chemoradiation when compared with surgery alone or surgery plus radiation. Although most preoperative radiation trials showed reductions in local relapse with the addition of preoperative radiation to surgical resection, only a large Swedish trial showed increased OS when compared to surgery alone.

Ongoing randomized trials will assess optimal combinations of postoperative chemoradiation (US GI Intergroup) and sequencing issues of pre-operative versus postoperative chemoradiation (Germany trial), and determine whether or not concurrent and maintenance 5-FU and leucovorin add to the benefits found with preoperative radiation (European Organization for Research and Treatment of Cancer).

A randomized trial has not yet been completed comparing chemoradiation to radiotherapy alone in the preoperative setting. The rationale for concurrent chemoradiotherapy is based on extrapolation from postoperative trials.

The success of combined modality chemotherapy and radiation in the adjuvant setting led to increased interest in this approach in the neoadjuvant setting. Phase II studies have demonstrated higher rates of pathological complete response (pCR) after chemoradiotherapy compared to series using radiation therapy alone. After moderate to high-dose preoperative radiation alone, pCR was found in 6 to 12% of patients, whereas 5-FU-based chemotherapy regimens combined with radiation showed pCR rates of 15 to 37%. Current guidelines from the National Comprehensive

Cancer Network recommend consideration of neoadjuvant chemoradiation for patients with T_3 or T_4 tumors.

Three randomized trials of preoperative versus postoperative combined-modality therapy for clinically respectable, T_3 rectal cancer, have been undertaken. The two American studies, NSABPR-03 and Intergroup 0147, closed early due to inadequate accrual; however, a preliminary analysis from the NSABP R-03 trial supports the use of preoperative treatment: 23% of patients in the preoperative arm had a complete clinical response (44% were pathologically confirmed), and preoperative therapy was associated with a higher rate of DFS compared to the postoperative treatment arm (DFS, 83% vs 78%) that did not reach statistical significance, and a higher rate of DFS with an intact sphincter (44% vs 34%). The rate of postoperative complications was similar between groups. The rate of grade 4 diarrhea during treatment, however, was significantly higher in the preoperative treatment group (24% vs 12%).

A third trial comparing preoperative versus postoperative chemoradiation, German trial CAO/ARO/AIO 94, completed accrual of over 800 patients with clinically staged T_3 or T_4 or node-positive rectal cancer. All patients received the same chemoradiation regimen, either preoperatively or postoperatively (with 5-FU daily for 5 days during the first and fifth week of radiation). All patients had surgery, including TME, and received four additional cycles of adjuvant single-agent 5-FU. In a preliminary report with 43-month median follow-up, preoperative chemoradiation was associated with a significantly lower pelvic relapse rate (7% vs 11%). The DFS and OS rates were similar. Significant downstaging of tumor was seen in the preoperative group, and patients in the preoperative treatment arm were twice as likely to undergo a sphincter-sparing surgery (39% vs 19%). Toxicity rates were similar in both treatment arms; however, patients undergoing neoadjuvant therapy had a decreased incidence of anastomotic strictures.

Surgery should be performed 4 to 7 weeks after completion of radiation. This delay allows time for recovery from the acute side effects of radiation and adequate time for tumor downstaging. Data from the Lyon R90-01 trial of preoperative radiation suggests that an interval of more than 2 weeks after the completion of radiation increased tumor downstaging. The incidence of sphincter preservation in this trial was 44%. Other series of Phase I/II trials for preoperative therapy in patients with clinically resectable rectal cancer have reported rates from 66 to 89%.

Although 5-FU is the standard chemotherapeutic agent used concurrently with radiation therapy, newer chemotherapeutic agents, including capecitabine, irinotecan, and oxaliplatin, have also been studied as radiosensitizers; and novel targeted biological agents are being explored in combination with standard chemotherapy and radiation therapy.

Clinical Pearls

1. Rectal cancer more frequently presents with symptoms than colon cancer and is more often associated with rectal bleeding (though less often with anemia).

2. Clinical staging is essential and includes physical exam, CT scan, rectal ultrasound, and, increasingly, MRI.

3. Neoadjuvant chemoradiation (using either infusional or bolus 5-FU and leucovorin) is increasingly being used for clinical stage T_3 or T_4 rectal cancers to downstage tumor and attempt sphincter-preserving surgery.

REFERENCES

1. Brown G, Davies S, Williams GT, et al: Effectiveness of preoperative staging in rectal cancer: Digital rectal examination, endoluminal ultrasound or magnetic resonance imaging? Br J Ca 91:23-29, 2004.
2. Jemal A, Tiwari RC, Murray T, et al: Cancer statistics, 2004. CA Cancer J Clin 54:8, 2004.
3. Crane C, Skibber J: Preoperative chemoradiation for locally advanced rectal cancer: Rationale, technique and results of treatment. Semin Surg Oncol 21:265-270, 2003.
4. Gunderson LL, Haddock MG, Schild SE: Rectal cancer: Preoperative versus postoperative irradiation as a component of adjuvant treatment. Semin Radiat Oncol 13(4):419-432, 2003.
5. Sauer R, Becker H, Hohenberger W: Adjuvant versus neoadjuvant combined modality treatment for locally advanced rectal cancer: First results of the German Rectal Cancer Study (CAO/ARO/AIO-94) (abstract). Int J Radiat Oncol Biol Phys 57:S124, 2003.
6. Hiotis SP, Weber SM, Cohen AM, et al: Assessing the predictive value of clinical complete response to neoadjuvant therapy for rectal cancer: An analysis of 488 patients. J Am Coll Surg 194:131, 2002.
7. Greene FL, Page DL, Fleming IL, et al (eds): AJCC (American Joint Committee on Cancer) Cancer Staging Manual, 6th ed., New York, Springer-Verlag, 2002, p 114.
8. Minsky BD: Sphincter preservation for rectal cancer: Fact or fiction? J Clin Oncol 20:1971, 2002.

9. Adjuvant radiotherapy for rectal cancer: A systemic overview of 8507 patients from 22 randomised trials. Colorectal Cancer Collaborative Group. Lancet 358:1291, 2001.

10. Grann A, Feng C, Wong D, et al: Preoperative combined modality therapy for clinically resectable uT3 rectal adenocarcinoma. Int J Radiat Oncol Biol Phys 49:987-995, 2001.

11. Roh MS, Petrelli N, Weiand H, et al: Phase III randomized trial of preoperative versus postoperative multimodality therapy in patients with carcinoma of the rectum (NSABP R-03). Proc Am Soc Clin Oncol 20:123a (Abstr 490), 2001.

12. Sauer R, Fietkau R, Wittekind C, et al: Adjuvant versus neoadjuvant radiochemotherapy for locally advanced rectal cancer. Strahlenther Onkol 177:173-181, 2001.

13. Camma C, Giunta M, Fiorica F, Pagliaro L: Preoperative radiotherapy for resectable rectal cancer: A meta-analysis. JAMA 284:1008, 2000.

14. Francois Y, Nemoz CJ, Baulieux J, et al: Influence of the interval between preoperative radiation therapy and surgery on downstaging and on the rate of sphincter-sparing surgery for rectal cancer: The Lyon R90-01 randomized trial. J Clin Oncol 17:2396-2402, 1999.

15. Improved survival with preoperative radiotherapy in resectable rectal cancer. Swedish Rectal Cancer Trial. N Engl J Med 336(14):980-987, 1997.

16. Hyams DM, Mamounas EP, Petrellli N, et al: A clinical trial to evaluate the worth of preoperative multimodality therapy in patients with operable carcinoma of the rectum: A progress report of National Surgical Breast and Bowel Project Protocol R-03. Dis Colon Rectum 40:131, 1997.

PATIENT 34

A 56-year-old man with metastatic colon carcinoma to the liver

A 56-year-old man has a history of stage III colon carcinoma, which was treated with a right hemicolectomy and adjuvant 5-FU/leucovorin 2 years ago. He is now found to have a solitary liver metastases on a follow-up CT scan of the abdomen. The patient is otherwise in good health and is asymptomatic.

Physical Examination: General: well-appearing, well-nourished. Vitals: stable. HEENT: anicteric. Lymph nodes: no palpable peripheral adenopathy. Cardiac: regular rate and rhythm. Abdomen: soft, nontender, with no hepatomegaly. Extremities: no clubbing, cyanosis, or edema.

Laboratory Findings: CBC: normal. Comprehensive panel: normal. CEA: 4.7 ng/mL. CT abdomen: new 2.7-cm solitary mass in right posterior-inferior lobe of liver (see Figure). FDG PET scan: avid uptake in right hepatic lobe lesion.

Question: What management options are available to this patient?

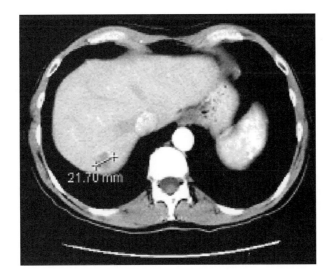

Answer: Surgical resection for solitary liver metastases is a curative option for this patient. Following hepatic resection, placement of a hepatic arterial infusion pump to deliver floxuridine (FUDR) locally along with systemic chemotherapy is a treatment option.

Discussion: The liver is the primary site of metastases for many patients with a variety of malignant neoplasms. Gastrointestinal tumors are particularly prone to spread to the liver because of portal venous drainage. In colorectal cancer, approximately 60% of patients will go on to develop hepatic metastases, and, in about one third, it will be the sole site of metastatic disease. In the setting of isolated liver metastases from colorectal cancer, significant progress has been made in the areas of hepatic resection, local ablative therapy, and regional chemotherapy.

In the United States, there are more than 50,000 patients a year with liver metastases from colorectal cancer. Resection of these metastases has been increasing as a result of several advances in hepatic surgery and because of expanding patient eligibility criteria. For patients undergoing liver resection, poor prognostic factors have been described in two large trials. The retrospective series from Memorial Sloan Kettering reviewed their experience with liver resections in 1001 patients with colorectal metastases from 1985 to 1998. The operative mortality was 2.8%, and 3-, 4-, and 5-year survival was 89%, 57%, and 37%, respectively. The number of tumors removed (greater or equal to 1), the size of the tumor removed (greater or less than 5 cm), the preoperative CEA level (greater or less than 200 ng/mL), the extent of resection (less than or greater than a lobectomy), the resection margin in the hepatic specimen (negative or positive), and the presence of extrahepatic disease were all highly significant predictors of postsurgical survival. A Clinical Risk Score (CRS) was devised from these data, using five clinical criteria: nodal status of the primary colorectal cancer, disease-free interval of less than 12 months, more than one tumor, prehepatic resection CEA level, and tumor size. Each risk factor was awarded one point, if the inferior condition existed, and points were added together to give the score. The 5-year survival for CRS of zero was 60% versus 14% survival for a score of 5.

Despite the high cure rate following hepatic resection, 75% of patients will experience recurrent metastases within 2 years, with approximately 50% recurring in the liver due to microscopic residual disease undetected at the time of resection. Although extrahepatic failure is of concern, the liver remains the predominant site of relapse, hence the rational for regional adjuvant chemotherapy. The use of hepatic artery infusion (HAI) chemotherapy after liver resection has been studied in a number of trials.

One such trial by Kemeny and colleagues reported the results of a randomized study of HAI fluorodeoxyuridine (FUDR) plus dexamethasone and systemic administration of 5-FU with or without leucovorin (LV) compared with systemic chemotherapy alone after the resection of hepatic metastases. The end points of the study were overall survival, survival free of hepatic progression, and overall progression-free survival at 2 years. The study enrolled 156 patients, and 20% had more than four hepatic lesions. Treatment in the combined modality arm consisted of 5-FU 320 mg/m^2 and LV 200 mg/m^2 followed by HAI FUDR and dexamethasone, initiated 2 weeks after the first cycle of 5-FU. Patients received pump infusion for 14 days, after which the pump was emptied and the patient was given 1 week of rest. In the systemic treatment group, 5-fluorouracil was administered at 375 mg/m^2 with the same dose of leucovorin for 5 days every 4 weeks. A total of six cycles were scheduled for each group. In patients previously treated with 5-FU and LV, 5-FU was administered as a continuous infusion at a dose of 850 mg/m^2 in the HAI group and 1000 mg/m^2 in the systemic group. Patients were stratified according to the number of liver metastases and type of previous chemotherapy.

Survival at 2 years was significantly increased with combined modality therapy (86% vs 72%, p = 0.03). Multivariate analysis showed an unadjusted risk ratio of 2.13 for death in the systemic group compared with the HAI plus systemic therapy group. Additionally, increased survival was seen with the HAI plus systemic therapy group of 72.2 months as opposed to 59.3 months in the systemic therapy group. Hepatic recurrence was also much decreased in the patients treated with HAI plus systemic therapy. Overall progression-free survival was also better with the HAI plus systemic therapy arm, with 57% free of progression at 2 years compared to 42% in the systemic therapy arm. Toxicity was increased in the combined group with increased diarrhea and increased liver function test abnormalities.

The Eastern Cooperative Oncology Group and Southwest Oncology Group conducted a prospective randomized multicenter trial of hepatic resection alone (group A) versus resection followed by four cycles of HAI with floxuridine and 12 cycles of systemic infusional 5-fluorouracil (group B). Only patients with three or fewer hepatic metastases from colorectal cancer were enrolled; 110 patients were randomized preoperatively, 56 in group A, and 54 in group B. A trend toward increased survival was seen with survival at 5 years reported as 32% in group A and 63% in group B. Three-year recurrence free rate was significantly greater with combined modality therapy versus resection alone, 58% and 34%, respectively (p = 0.039). In addition, less involvement of the liver with hepatic recurrence was noted in group B (8%) versus group A (24%), which was of statistical significance (p = 0.035).

Few trials have evaluated systemic chemotherapy alone as adjuvant therapy following hepatic resection for colorectal cancer. One study reported by Portier and colleagues randomized 173 patients to systemic therapy versus control after liver resection. At 5 years, progression-free survival was 32.2% versus 25.5%, p = 0.12. Overall survival at 5 years was 50% versus 40%, p = 0.15.

Following hepatic resection for colorectal cancer, systemic chemotherapy or HAI therapy with FUDR and systemic therapy is a reasonable option. As more agents become available for the treatment of colorectal cancer, it remains to be determined what the optimal adjuvant therapy should be for patients with resected hepatic metastases.

The present patient underwent a successful partial hepatectomy and placement of a hepatic arterial infusion pump. He tolerated 6 months of hepatic arterial FUDR therapy and systemic irinotecan on a clinical protocol. He remained free of disease for a year, and then the disease recurred in abdominal lymph nodes and lung. He is presently receiving additional systemic chemotherapy with oxaliplatin and 5-FU.

Clinical Pearls

1. In colorectal cancer, approximately 60% of patients will go on to develop hepatic metastases, and, in about one third, it will be the sole site of metastatic disease.

2. In the setting of isolated liver metastases from colorectal cancer, hepatic resection can be curative in select patients.

3. Despite the high cure rate following hepatic resection, 75% of patients will experience recurrent metastases within 2 years, with approximately 50% recurring in the liver.

4. Combined systemic chemotherapy and hepatic arterial infusion of FUDR therapy have been shown to decrease hepatic and extrahepatic rates of recurrence following resection of hepatic metastases.

REFERENCES

1. Cohen AD, Kemeny NE: An update on hepatic arterial infusion chemotherapy for colorectal cancer. The Oncologist 8:553-566, 2003.
2. Kemeny MM, Adak S, Gray B, et al: Combined-modality treatment for resectable metastatic colorectal carcinoma to the liver: Surgical resection of hepatic metastases in combination with continuous infusion of chemotherapy: An intergroup study. J Clin Oncol 20:1499-1505, 2002.
3. Kemeny N, Huang Y, Cohen AM, et al: Hepatic arterial infusion of chemotherapy after resection of hepatic metastases from colorectal cancer. N Engl J Med 341:2039-2048, 1999.

John Gerecitano, MD, PhD

PATIENT 35

A 75-year-old woman with abdominal pain and an abnormal colonic biopsy

A 75-year-old woman with a distant history of breast cancer presents with a 5-month history of abdominal pain, constipation, and bloating. Workup includes a mammogram showing fibrocystic changes, fine-needle aspirates of a mass in the left breast consistent with benign changes, a transvaginal ultrasound revealing no obvious masses, and a colonoscopy that revealed a 0.5-cm polyp. A colonoscopic biopsy is notable for poorly differentiated adenocarcinoma of the colonic mucosa, felt to be extrinsic in origin from the colon. Immunohistochemical staining is positive for CK7 and negative for CK20. A CT scan of the chest, abdomen, and pelvis shows linear markings consistent with metastases in the greater omentum, an increased number of subcentimeter left axillary lymph nodes, distal colonic wall thickening, and a thickened gallbladder wall.

Physical Examination: General: fatigued-appearing, no acute distress, weight 51 kg, height 145 cm. Vital signs: temperature 37.5°C, pulse 72, respiration 16, blood pressure 120/62. HEENT: no scleral icterus. Lymph nodes: two mobile lymph nodes in left axilla measuring 1 cm each. Breasts: 3-cm mobile round mass in left breast. Chest: clear bilaterally. Abdomen: soft, nontender, slightly distended, bowel sounds present. Extremities: no edema.

Laboratory Findings: Serum markers include CA-125 = 27.3, CA19-9 = 82, and CEA = 3.7.

Question: What additional tests should be ordered to establish the primary site of the patient's carcinoma?

Answer: Additional workup should include a review of pathology with additional staining, PET scan, and evaluation of the left breast by a surgeon.

Discussion: The cytokeratin profile of the patient's biopsy is not consistent with a primary colonic adenocarcinoma (less than 1% of these are CK7$^+$/CK20$^-$). Therefore, the patient may be diagnosed with carcinoma of unknown primary (CUP). CUPs represent approximately 2 to 5% of all invasive cancers diagnosed in the United States each year. More than 60% of CUPs are adenocarcinomas, and the primary sites are never identified in the majority of cases. Prognosis for CUP is poor, with a median survival of 6 to 9 months. However, there are several treatable subgroups that have a more favorable prognosis, for example, men with blastic bone metastases, women with peritoneal adenocarcinoma, squamous cell cancers of certain sites, and men with poorly differentiated carcinoma, with midline retroperitoneal disease.

Limit workup of patients with CUP and start empirical therapy, if no primary site is found after reasonable investigation. Clinical investigation should include a complete history and physical examination, chemistry profile, CBC, and radiograph and CT scan of the chest/abdomen/pelvis, along with appropriate radiological studies of symptomatic areas. Perform mammography in any woman with axillary adenopathy, and measure serum prostate-specific antigen (PSA) in men with blastic bone lesions. Serum human chorionic gonadotropin (hCG), alpha-fetoprotein (AFP), and lactate dehydrogenase should be determined in all young men with poorly differentiated carcinoma. A PET scan may help identify the primary site in a proportion of patients.

Cervical adenopathy involved with squamous cell carcinoma should prompt a full evaluation of the head and neck, including endoscopy with biopsies of the oropharynx, hypopharynx, nasopharynx, larynx, and upper esophagus. Inguinal adenopathy should prompt a thorough search of the perineal area. Tumor markers are not specific enough to be useful in establishing a diagnosis but can be followed to gauge effectiveness of treatment.

Pathological staining can help to identify the site of origin for some CUPs. Staining for PSA may identify metastatic prostate cancer in men, and stains for estrogen and progesterone receptors can identify breast carcinomas in women. Other stains to consider include leukocyte common antigen (anaplastic lymphoma), S100 (melanoma), neuron specific enolase, chromogranin and synaptophysin (neuroendocrine tumors), cytokeratin (carcinoma), vimentin and desmin (sarcoma), TK1 (thyroid, lung), placental alkaline phosphatase, hCG and AFP (germ cell tumors), HER-2 (breast), thyroglobulin, and calcitonin (thyroid). Electron microscopy can help distinguish ultrastructural features of lymphoma, carcinoma, melanoma, and neuroendocrine tumors. If germ cell tumor (GCT) is suspected, molecular pathology can confirm the status of i12p (highly sensitive for GCTs).

If a primary site is not evident after the previously described workup, initiate empirical treatment. Women with isolated axillary LAD should be treated for presumed stage II breast cancer, whereas those with peritoneal carcinomatosis should be treated for presumed stage III ovarian cancer. Men with blastic bone lesions and elevated PSA should be treated for prostate cancer, whereas young men with mediastinal or retroperitoneal masses should be treated for extragonadal GCT. If the tumor has neuroendocrine features, use a platinum/etoposide-based regimen. All other patients with good performance status should be treated with a platinum/etoposide-based regimen, such as that proposed by Greco and colleagues: paclitaxel 200 mg/m^2 plus carboplatin AUC = 6 once every 3 weeks, with etoposide 50 mg alternating with 100 mg per day on days 1 to 10. This regimen has achieved a response rate of 13%, median survival of 13.4 months, 2-year overall survival of 20%, and 4-year overall survival of 14%.

The present patient underwent an excisional biopsy of the dominant mass in her left breast. Pathological evaluation revealed an invasive lobular carcinoma. The patient was treated for metastatic breast cancer with anastrozole.

Clinical Pearls

1. In patients with carcinoma of unknown primary (CUP), a limited workup to identify a primary site is appropriate but should not unduly delay empirical treatment.

2. The clinical subtype of CUP should be identified to determine the type of empirical therapy. Currently available chemotherapeutic options for CUP have extended median survival of 3 to 4 months to 9 to 13 months.

3. The primary site of the tumor becomes obvious in only 15 to 20% of patients with CUP. Tumor markers are not generally useful in establishing a diagnosis

REFERENCES

1. Pavlidis N: Cancer of unknown primary: Biological and clinical characteristics. Ann Oncol 14(Suppl 3):iii11-iii18, 2003.
2. Hainsworth JD: Carcinoma of unknown primary site. In Pazdur R, Coia LR, Hoskins WJ, Wagman LD (eds.): Cancer Management: A Multidisciplinary Approach. New York, PRR Inc., 2002.
3. Tot T: Cytokeratins 20 and 7 as biomarkers: Usefulness in discriminating primary from metastatic adenocarcinoma. Eur J Cancer 38:758-763, 2002.

PATIENT 36

A 62-year-old man with dysphagia for solid food

A 62-year-old man with chronic dyspepsia notes a 35-pound weight loss over the past year. Recently, he has developed mild dysphagia for solid foods. He feels as though foods become stuck in the bottom of his throat. He denies any nausea, vomiting, abdominal pain, or changes in his stools.

Physical Examination: Temperature 37.1°C, blood pressure 137/84, pulse 104. HEENT: anicteric, oropharynx clear, no adenopathy. Cardiac: regular rate and rhythm. Chest: clear to auscultation. Abdomen: normal active bowel sounds, soft, nontender, nondistended, no organomegaly. Extremities: no cyanosis, clubbing, or edema.

Laboratory Findings: CBC: WBC 11,100/μL with normal differential, hemoglobin 10.4 g/dL, MCV 74, platelets 456,000/μL. Biochemistry profile: normal. Liver function tests: normal. Chest radiograph: normal. CT scan of abdomen: thickening in stomach wall along greater curvature without regional lymphadenopathy or liver lesions (see Figure). Endoscopy: 5.7 cm × 3.8 cm mass in antrum of stomach. Pathology from endoscopic biopsy: adenocarcinoma of proximal stomach.

Question: What is the appropriate management for nonmetastatic gastric adenocarcinoma?

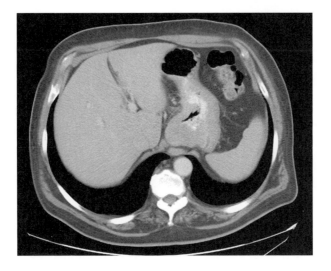

Answer: Surgical resection followed by adjuvant chemoradiation is recommended in the management of early-stage resectable gastric adenocarcinoma.

Discussion: There are approximately 21,000 new cases of gastric cancer in the United States each year. This disease is often unresectable at the time of diagnosis. Among those patients who undergo complete surgical resection, most will, ultimately, experience disease recurrence.

Complete surgical resection (an R0 resection) remains the basis for treatment with curative intent in gastric carcinoma. Success is highest when disease is identified early, with a 5-year survival for stage IA disease at 78 to 86% but less than 50% for stage II and above in Western countries.

Locoregional failure is a major site of recurrence following gastric resection with curative intent, especially for more deeply penetrating (T_3) tumors or those with lymph node metastases, although extra-abdominal spread without intra-abdominal metastases occurs rarely. The most common sites of intra-abdominal failure are regional and distant lymph node groups, peritoneal cavity, and liver. Herein lies the rationale for the consideration of multimodality therapy for the treatment of patients with gastric cancer beyond the earliest stages, including the use of adjuvant treatment. A previous description by Shah and Kelsen of disease recurrence management serves as the basis for the following discussion.

Prior to the publication of intergroup study 116 (INT-116) in 2001, postoperative chemotherapy and radiation were not firmly established as beneficial, particularly in studies that did not employ a multimodality approach. INT-116 was a large, randomized trial that tested the hypothesis that chemotherapy plus radiation therapy following curative intent resection of gastric carcinoma was superior to surgery alone. From 1991 to 1998, 556 patients with stage IB to IVA gastric or gastroesophageal junction adenocarcinomas were assigned randomly to receive either surgery alone or surgery followed by chemoradiotherapy. All patients underwent an R0 resection, 10% of patients underwent a D2 lymph-node dissection, and 36% of patients underwent a D1 dissection (removal of all N1 perigastric lymph nodes). Most patients underwent a D0 resection (54%), which is less than a complete dissection of the N1 lymph nodes.

Most patients were considered high risk for relapse (stage IIIA or IIIB by 1988 AJCC staging criteria), with 85% having lymph node involvement and over 67% with T_3 or T_4 tumors. Only 36 patients had stage IB disease. Most tumors were in the distal stomach, with 20% of patients having tumors that were located at the gastroesophageal junction.

Patients in the treatment arm first received chemotherapy with fluorouracil and leucovorin for 5 days. One month later, patients received chemotherapy-sensitized radiation. One month after completion of radiation, additional chemotherapy was administered for 2 additional months.

With a median follow-up of 5 years, the median survival and overall 3-year survival rate for the chemoradiotherapy group was 36 months and 50% and, for the surgery-only group, 27 months and 41%, respectively (p = 0.005). The median duration of relapse-free survival was 30 months in the chemoradiotherapy group and 19 months in the surgery-only group (p < 0.001). Relapses occurred in 64% of patients in the surgery-only group and in 43% of the patients who were assigned to the chemoradiotherapy arm. Patients treated with surgery only were more likely to experience local and regional recurrence than were patients who received adjuvant chemoradiation. Distant relapse was more common in the chemoradiation arm (32 patients, 18%) than in the surgery-only arm (40 patients, 33%).

The adjuvant therapy was moderately toxic, with 54% of patients developing significant (i.e., grade 3 or higher) hematological toxicity and 33% complaining of significant gastrointestinal symptoms. There were three treatment-related deaths (1%). The planned therapy was completed by 181 patients (64%). The primary reasons for not completing therapy were due to toxicity (49 patients, 17%) or patient withdrawal (23 patients, 8%).

These data support the use of chemoradiation therapy after surgical resection for gastric cancer patients with stages II, IIIA, and IIIB. Although there are concerns regarding the extent of surgical resection performed in this trial, the analysis does not suggest an influence of type of dissection on survival.

In the United States, only 31% of patients undergo an R0 resection, meaning that this study applies to approximately 7000 American patients annually. Strategies to improve the R0 resection rate are needed. Currently, the use of preoperative chemotherapy or chemoradiation is under active investigation. Postoperative intraperitoneal therapy is also being evaluated to decrease the risk of peritoneal failure. Finally, there are data to suggest that better systemic chemotherapy may be available in the near future, with the use of such agents as docetaxel, paclitaxel, and irinotecan.

The present patient has been scheduled for a surgical resection with an eye toward adjuvant chemoradiation.

Clinical Pearls

1. In resectable gastric adenocarcinoma, adjuvant chemoradiation appears to confer a significant improvement in overall survival.
2. The optimal extent of lymph node dissection during surgery remains controversial.

REFERENCES

1. Shah MA, Kelsen DP: Postoperative adjuvant chemoradiotherapy in high risk gastric cancer. Chirurg 73(4):325-330, 2002.
2. Macdonald JS, Smalley SR, Benedetti J, et al: Chemoradiotherapy after surgery compared with surgery alone for adenocarcinoma of the stomach or gastroesophageal junction. N Engl J Med 345(10):725-730, 2001.
3. Hundahl S, Phillips J, Menck H: The National Cancer Data Base Report on Poor Survival of U.S. Gastric Carcinoma Patients Treated with Gastrectomy, 5th ed. American Joint Committee on Cancer—Staging, proximal disease, and the "different disease" hypothesis. Cancer 88:921-932, 2000.
4. Mari E, Floriani I, Tinazzi A, et al: Efficacy of adjuvant chemotherapy after curative resection for gastric cancer: A meta-analysis of published randomized trials. Ann Oncol 11:837-843, 2000.
5. Earle CC, Maroun JA: Adjuvant chemotherapy after curative resection for gastric cancer in non-Asian patients: Revisiting a meta-analysis of randomized trials. Eur J Cancer 37:1059-1064, 1999.
6. Roder JD, Bottcher K, Busch R, et al: Classification of regional lymph node metastasis from gastric carcinoma. Cancer 82:621-631, 1998.
7. Hallissey MT, Dunn JA, Ward LC, Allum WH: The second British Cancer Group trial of adjuvant radiotherapy or chemotherapy in resectable gastric cancer: Five-year follow-up. Lancet 343:1309-1312, 1994.

PATIENT 37

A 66-year-old man with newly diagnosed metastatic gastric cancer

A 66-year-old man with a history of a Billroth II procedure for peptic ulcer disease presents to his primary physician with a 4-month history of intermittent abdominal pain, fatigue, and 85-pound weight loss. The patient's symptoms progressed to frequent nausea and vomiting over the past 2 weeks. Endoscopy demonstrated an 8 cm × 5 cm ulcerated mass lesion in his stomach, extending from the proximal lesser curvature to the posterior wall.

Physical Examination: Temperature 37.2°C, pulse 86, blood pressure 140/80. General: obese. HEENT: sclerae anicteric, dry mucous membranes. Abdomen: moderate epigastric tenderness is present, no shifting dullness. Extremities: no edema.

Laboratory Findings: Biopsy from gastric mass: invasive, poorly differentiated adenocarcinoma. Biochemistry profile: electrolytes normal. BUN 8, creatinine 1.1. CT scan of chest, abdomen (see Figure), and pelvis: mediastinal and hilar lymphadenopathy; numerous pulmonary nodules; ascites; numerous perigastric, splenic hilum; gastrohepatic; and celiac lymph nodes are present.

Question: What treatment options are available for metastatic gastric cancer?

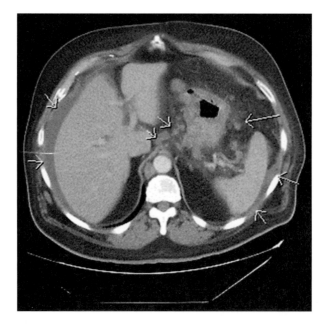

Answer: Cisplatin-based chemotherapy is the treatment of choice in patients with metastatic gastric cancer.

Discussion: Gastric cancer is the second most common cancer worldwide after lung cancer. The disease is most prevalent in Japan, Chile, and Scandinavia. In the United States, there are approximately 22,000 new cases of gastric cancer a year. At presentation, 80% of patients have advanced inoperable disease. For these patients, chemotherapy is a useful palliative option that has been demonstrated to improve median survival when compared to "best supportive care." Several single-agent chemotherapy drugs have been studied in advanced gastric cancer (see Table 1). These agents result in a response rate of 8 to 30%. Responses are generally incomplete and of short duration.

The low therapeutic activity of single-agent chemotherapy has led to the development of combination regimens. Combination chemotherapy results in higher responses and longer median survival. In phase II trials of some common combinations, such as FAMTX (fluorouracil, doxorubicin, high-dose methotrexate), ECF (epirubicin, cisplatin, fluorouracil), ELF (etoposide, leucovorin, fluorouracil), and CF (cisplatin, fluorouracil), response rates range from 20 to 60%. Several randomized trials have been performed, in an attempt to define the most superior regimen in metastatic gastric carcinoma (see Table 2). There remains considerable debate as to which regimen is the best, but many investigators agree that cisplatin and fluorouracil-based therapy is a standard reference regimen. Another front-line regimen is weekly irinotecan with cisplatin. In phase II trials, this regimen results in response rates of 30 to 60%. In the UK and Europe, ECF is the preferred regimen. Researchers at MD Anderson Cancer Center have been instrumental in incorporating docetaxel into the treatment regimen for metastatic gastric cancer. Their favored first-line regimen is DCF (docetaxel, cisplatin, fluorouracil), which has been shown to produce significant improvements in response rate and time to progression in an interim analysis. However, this regimen is very toxic, with 84% of patients developing grade 3 or 4 neutropenia, and 68% developing nonhematological grade 3 or 4 adverse events. Concerns about the toxicity of this regimen have limited its general use in the oncology community.

The present patient was treated with irinotecan and cisplatin combination chemotherapy. He achieved a good partial response that was maintained for 6 months. His disease, subsequently, progressed and did not respond to second-line chemotherapy.

Table 1. Response Rates of Single-Agent Chemotherapy in Advanced Gastric Cancer

Agent	Patients	Response (%)
5-FU	416	21
Cisplatin	139	19
Doxorubicin	221	18
Mitomycin	211	30
UFT	188	28
Carboplatin	41	8
Paclitaxel	55	11
Docetaxel	86	20
Irinotecan	60	23
VP-16	26	17

5-FU = 5-fluorouracil; UFT = Tegafur-Uracil; VP-16 = etoposide.

Table 2. Combination Chemotherapy Trials for Advanced Gastric and Gastroesophageal Junction Carcinoma

Agents	Patients	Response (%)	Median Survival (mo)
ELF vs	245	9	7.2
FAMTX vs		12	6.7
CF		20	7.2
FAMTX vs	274	21	6.1
ECF		46	8.7
MCF vs	580	44	8.7
ECF		42	9.4
DC vs	148	23	8.5
DCF		39	10.2

ELF = epirubicin, cisplatin, fluorouracil; FAMTX = fluorouracil, doxorubicin, high-dose methotrexate; CF = cisplatin, fluorouracil; ECF = epirubicin, cisplatin, fluorouracil; MCF = mitomycin, cisplatin, fluorouracil; DC = docetaxel, cisplatin; DCF = docetaxel, cisplatin, fluorouracil.

Clinical Pearls

1. There are approximately 22,000 new cases of gastric cancer a year in the United States. At presentation, 80% of patients have advanced inoperable disease.

2. Cisplatin and fluorouracil-based therapy is the standard palliative regimen for metastatic gastric cancer. Taxanes and epirubicin have been successfully incorporated into first-line therapy with cisplatin and 5-FU; however, because of significant toxicity, these newer regimens have not been widely adopted.

REFERENCES

1. Shah MA, Schwartz GK: Treatment of metastatic esophagus and gastric cancer. Semin Oncol 31(4):574-587, 2004.
2. Murad AM: Chemotherapy for advanced gastric cancer: Focus on new agents and combinations. Cancer Control 6(4): 361-368, 1999.
3. Fuchs CS, Mayer RJ: Gastric carcinoma. N Engl J Med 333:32-41, 1995.

PATIENT 38

A 60-year-old man with dysphagia and odynophagia

A 60-year-old man with a history of chronic heartburn and heavy alcohol and tobacco use presents to a gastroenterologist with a 4-week history of progressive dysphagia and odynophagia. Endoscopy reveals a fungating mass at the gastroesophageal (GE) junction. A biopsy is consistent with poorly differentiated adenocarcinoma. He is referred to an oncologist's office for further recommendations.

Physical Examination: General: thin, no acute distress. Temperature 36.9°C, blood pressure 110/60 mmHg, pulse 92, weight 73 kg. HEENT: anicteric sclerae, oral mucosa moist without lesions, no lymphadenopathy, hearing exam normal. Cardiac: regular rate and rhythm, with no murmurs. Chest: clear to auscultation bilaterally. Abdomen: nontender, nondistended, active bowel sounds. Extremities: no edema.

Laboratory Findings: Electrolytes, complete blood count, and transaminases: normal. CT scan of chest and abdomen: esophageal thickening extending from carina to GE junction with slight narrowing of esophageal lumen; bulky lymphadenopathy in mediastinum, subcarinal region, and right hilum; two hypodense masses in right liver lobe consistent with metastatic disease. PET scan: increased uptake at the primary tumor, liver lesions, and mediastinal lymph nodes.

Questions: What is the most likely diagnosis? What treatment is indicated?

Answers: Metastatic esophageal cancer. Palliative chemotherapy is recommended.

Discussion: Esophageal cancers are relatively rare in the United States (fewer than 5 in 100,000) but are more common worldwide, particularly in China and the former Soviet republics. Tobacco and ethanol exposure are believed to be the principal risk factors in the United States, whereas dietary practices may be more contributory in Asia. It remains controversial whether Barrett's esophagus—a condition characterized by the proliferation of columnar epithelium in the distal esophagus, likely caused by chronic acid reflux—is a risk factor for esophageal cancer.

The most common types of esophagus cancer are squamous cell and adenocarcinoma. The incidence of adenocarcinoma has been steadily rising in the United States, whereas the rate of squamous cell cancer has remained stable. Generally, these tumor types are treated similarly. Other rare subtypes include small cell tumors and sarcomas.

Evaluation for esophageal cancer involves direct evaluation with endoscopy and biopsy. Staging workup should include a CT scan of the chest and abdomen to assess for the presence of locoregional lymph nodes or distant spread (most commonly in the liver). Accurate staging is vital to avoid potentially morbid surgical or radiation therapies in those with metastatic disease, such as this patient.

The American Joint Committee on Cancer (AJCC) staging of esophageal cancer utilizes TNM criteria, with prognosis related directly to stage. At the time of diagnosis, approximately half of patients have metastatic disease and are candidates for palliative management. For local control of dysphagia, esophageal dilation, radiation, or endoscopically-placed stents may be used. Single-agent or multi-agent chemotherapy regimens have been evaluated, with reported responses in 15 to 60% of patients. Multiple agents are reported to possess activity, including platinum drugs, topoisomerase inhibitors, fluorouracil, taxanes, and vinorelbine.

A combination of cisplatin and irinotecan given weekly has been associated with responses in 51 to 66% of patients, leading to improved dysphagia and quality of life. Cisplatin and infusional fluorouracil remain common first-line agents for metastatic disease, although regimens including irinotecan or taxanes appear to mediate higher response rates. Recent phase III trials suggest that adding epirubicin or docetaxel to fluorouracil/cisplatin may increase rates of response and survival. Nonetheless, duration of response is usually brief, with a median survival of less than 1 year even with chemotherapy.

The present patient began treatment with weekly combination cisplatin/irinotecan. Initial follow-up CT scan showed a 30% reduction in the size of his liver lesions.

Clinical Pearls

1. Metastatic esophageal cancer is treated with palliative chemotherapy. Multiple agents have been evaluated and appear to possess activity.

2. Local measures for control of dysphagia may be required, such as esophageal stenting, dilation, or radiation.

3. Duration of response to palliative chemotherapy is often brief, with median survival of less than 1 year.

REFERENCES

1. Allum W, Cunningham D, Weeden S (National Cancer Research Institute Upper Gastrointestinal Clinical Study Group): Perioperative chemotherapy in operable gastric and lower esophageal cancer: A randomised controlled trial (the MAGIC trial ISRCTN 93793971). Proc Am Soc Clin Oncol 21:998, 2003.
2. Siewert JR, Stein HJ, Sendler A, et al: Esophageal cancer: Clinical management. In Kelsen DP, Daly JM, Kern SE, et al (eds): Gastrointestinal Oncology: Principles and Practice. Philadelphia, Lippincott Williams & Wilkins, 2002, pp 261-287.
3. Ajani J, Fairwhether J, Pisters P: MD Anderson Center: Phase II study of CPT-11 plus cisplatin in patients with advanced gastric and GE junction carcinomas. Proc Am Soc Clin Oncol 18:241, 1999.
4. Blot WJ, McLaughlin JK: The changing epidemiology of esophageal cancer. Semin Oncol 26:2, 1999.
5. Ilson DH, Saltz L, Enzinger P: Phase II trial of weekly irinotecan plus cisplatin in advanced esophageal cancer. J Clin Oncol 17:3270, 1999.

PATIENT 39

A 69-year-old woman with abdominal pain

A 69-year-old woman with a remote history of stage I infiltrating lobular carcinoma of the breast presents with severe mid-epigastric abdominal pain, loss of appetite, and diminished energy.

Physical Examination: General: thin, well-appearing. Temperature 37°C, blood pressure 110/70 mmHg, pulse 100, weight 54 kg. HEENT: sclerae anicteric, no pallor, no lymphadenopathy. Cardiac: regular rate and rhythm, with no murmurs. Chest: clear to auscultation bilaterally. Abdomen: epigastric fullness with a barely palpable supraumbilical mass, mildly tender hepatomegaly, active bowel sounds, no ascites. Extremities: no edema.

Laboratory Findings: Electrolytes: normal. AST 48, ALT 51, alkaline phosphatase 263, total bilirubin 0.6, albumin 3.0, LDH 577, CEA 122.5, CA 19-9 830. CT scan of abdomen: multiple lesions in the liver, a 4.7-cm mass in the tail of the pancreas, and multiple small bilateral pulmonary nodules. CT-guided biopsy of liver: metastatic moderately differentiated adenocarcinoma, favoring a pancreatic primary. These slides are compared to the patient's breast cancer slides and are felt to be histologically dissimilar.

Question: What is the recommended treatment for this patient?

Answer: Systemic chemotherapy for metastatic pancreatic cancer is the recommended treatment.

Discussion: The patient has pancreatic cancer that is already metastatic at the time of diagnosis. Therefore, she is not a surgical candidate, and systemic treatment in the form of chemotherapy is indicated. Since 1997, gemcitabine has been first-line treatment for pancreatic cancer, with improved clinical outcomes, including decreased pain and improved performance status when compared to 5-fluorouracil. In addition, gemcitabine yields a longer average time to progression and improved 12-month survival than 5-fluorouracil.

However, response rates and overall survival remain dismal. Current clinical trials are examining the role of agents to be used in combination with gemcitabine, such as cisplatin and oxaliplatin. Based on favorable preliminary data, this patient was treated with gemcitabine in combination with cisplatin. After three cycles of this regimen, a CT scan documented decreased size of her pancreatic, lung, and liver lesions. She received an additional three cycles of gemcitabine and cisplatin, but subsequent reimaging demonstrated a marked increase in the size of her liver lesions and multiple new bilateral pulmonary emboli (the risk of thrombotic events in pancreatic cancer is particularly high, and prophylactic anticoagulation has been proposed by some, although this area remains controversial with limited available data).

A growing number of familial syndromes and specific genetic mutations have been associated with pancreatic cancer, including hereditary pancreatitis, hereditary nonpolyposis colon cancer (HNPCC), hereditary breast-ovarian cancer syndrome (via the BRCA2 gene), familial adenomatous polyposis, Peutz-Jeghers syndrome, and familial atypical multiple mole melanoma syndrome (FAMMM). The National Familial Pancreatic Tumor Registry has identified an increased risk for the development of pancreatic cancer in patients with one or more relatives diagnosed with this disease. However, there are no widely accepted screening strategies for pancreatic cancer at this time.

Clinical Pearls

1. Systemic chemotherapy with gemcitabine is considered first-line treatment for metastatic pancreatic cancer. The addition of other agents, such as platinum drugs, is under investigation.

2. The incidence of thrombotic events is particularly high in patients with pancreatic cancer.

REFERENCE

Burris HA III, Moore MJ, Andersen J, et al: Improvements in survival and clinical benefit with gemcitabine as first-line therapy for patients with advanced pancreas cancer: A randomized trial. J Clin Oncol 15:2403-2413, 1997.

PATIENT 40

A 66-year-old woman with obstructive jaundice

A 66-year-old woman presents with jaundice (bilirubin 8 mg/dL), dark urine, pale stools, and pruritus. A CT scan demonstrates a mass in the head of the pancreas with dilated bile and pancreatic ducts. Cytological evaluation of Endoscopic Retrograde Cholangiopancreatography (ERCP) brushings confirm pancreatic carcinoma. Whipple surgery reveals a 2.8 cm × 2.5 cm head of pancreas mass consistent with well to moderately differentiated adenocarcinoma. There is focal extension to the peripancreatic fat and perineural invasion, and 3/22 lymph nodes are positive for tumor. All margins are clear. The pathological stage is $T_3N_1M_0$, or stage IIB. The patient now seeks an opinion on the role of adjuvant therapy from medical oncology.

Physical Examination: General: well-appearing. Vitals: blood pressure 120/73 mmHg, pulse 91, temperature 36.6°C, respirations 20. HEENT: no scleral icterus, no lymphadenopathy. Chest: clear to auscultation bilaterally. Cardiovascular: regular rate and rhythm with no murmurs. Abdomen: soft, nontender, no masses, surgical scar present. Extremities: unremarkable. Neurological: normal.

Laboratory Findings: All normal.

Questions: Should the patient receive adjuvant therapy? If yes, what type of adjuvant therapy? If the patient were node-negative, would this change your treatment recommendations?

Answers: This patient should receive adjuvant therapy. In the United States, a controversial standard of care would be to use adjuvant chemoradiation, although clinical trials evaluating adjuvant therapy for resected pancreatic cancer have had conflicting results. Adjuvant therapy is recommended in the United States, irrespective of lymph node status.

Discussion: Using the sixth edition American Joint Committee on Cancer (AJCC) staging guidelines, the patient has pathological stage IIB (using the old system, the patient would have been classified as stage III) pancreatic cancer. In patients with locoregional pancreatic cancer, surgery provides the best chance for long-term survival; therefore, performing a Whipple resection in this patient was appropriate.

However, the optimal postoperative management of the patient is more contentious. In the United States the standard of care for adjuvant therapy for pancreatic cancer is chemoradiation. This treatment approach is based on the results of the first prospective randomized phase III trial, performed by the Gastrointestinal Tumor Study Group (GITSG), evaluating surgery and chemoradiation (500 mg/m^2/day of 5-FU for 6 days with 2 weeks of 40 Gy of radiation followed by weekly 5-FU alone for 2 years) versus surgery alone in 43 patients with locally advanced pancreatic cancer (see Table). This trial demonstrated a survival advantage for adjuvant chemoradiation therapy over surgery alone (median survival 21 months vs 10.9 months, p = 0.03). GITSG, subsequently, registered another 30 patients to receive adjuvant chemoradiation, and their median survival of 18 months supported the efficacy of adjuvant chemoradiation therapy.

Two other large studies have failed to replicate the results of the GITSG trial and are limited by their trial design. The European Organization for Research and Treatment of Cancer (EORTC) trial randomized 218 patients to surgery and chemoradiation (25 mg/kg/day continuous infusion 5-FU with 4 weeks of 40 Gy split course radiation) or surgery alone. There was a trend toward an improved median survival with the addition of chemoradiation (17 months vs 12.6 months), but

it was not statistically significant (p = 0.208). Although the authors concluded that adjuvant therapy should not be considered a standard of care, the results of this trial may be affected by inadequate power, lack of post-chemoradiation chemotherapy, exclusion of T$_3$ lesions, and the fact that 20% of patients in the chemoradiation group were treated by surgery alone.

The European Study Group for Pancreatic Cancer (ESPAC) randomized patients into a 2 × 2 factorial design (observation, chemoradiotherapy alone, chemotherapy alone, or both) or into one of the main treatment comparisons (chemoradiotherapy vs no chemoradiotherapy or chemotherapy vs no chemotherapy). The results from the 2 × 2 factorial design randomization have recently been updated. Unlike the GITSG and EORTC trials, patients in this trial could have positive tumor margins. Results from 541 eligible patients showed no benefit in median survival for the 175 patients in the chemoradiotherapy arm compared to the 178 patients in the "no chemoradiotherapy" arm (15.5 months vs 16.1 months, p = 0.24), but there was an improvement in median survival for the 238 patients who received chemotherapy compared to the 235 patients who did not receive chemotherapy (19.7 months vs 14 months), which was statistically significant (p = 0.0005). However, this trial also contains flaws—including a lack of standardized radiation technique, positive tumor margins, protocol violations, and the confounding effect of coexistent treatments. Due to the difficulty in interpreting the European trials, and based upon the positive results from the GITSG trial, chemoradiation remains the standard of care in the United States. Recent improvements in radiation techniques and chemotherapy add further support to the rationale for using adjuvant chemoradiation.

Randomized Studies of Chemoradiotherapy versus No Chemoradiotherapy

	Year of Study	Number of Patients	Actuarial Survival	Median Survival (mo)	p Value
GITSG	1985[1,2]	43	43% vs 18% (2 yr)	21 vs 10.9	0.03
Bakkevold et al	1993[7]	61	4% vs 8% (5 yr)	23 vs 11.4	0.02
EORTC	1999[3]	218	51% vs 41% (2 yr)	17 vs 12.6	0.208
ESPAC*	2001[4]	353	NR	15.5 vs 16.1	0.24

*2 × 2 factorial design; a statistically significant survival advantage was seen for the adjuvant chemotherapy arm compared to the "no chemotherapy" arm (median survival 19.7 months vs 14 months, p < .001).
NR = not reported.

Patients with both node-negative and node-positive disease were included in the randomized trials evaluating adjuvant therapy for pancreatic cancer, and thus the conclusion that chemoradiation is beneficial can apply to both node-negative and node-positive patients. Because the overall survival for patients with node-negative disease is better than node-positive cancer, one might expect node-negative patients to derive a greater benefit from chemoradiation because many patients with bulky node-positive tumors probably already have microscopic disease dissemination. In the ESPAC trial, stratification of the chemoradiotherapy and chemotherapy treatment comparisons by lymph-node status did not change the overall results seen.

Current studies by the Radiation Therapy Oncology Group (RTOG) and the ESPAC groups are evaluating gemcitabine as adjuvant therapy. The RTOG trial has two treatment arms containing infusional 5-fluorouracil with radiation with infusional 5-FU given before and after chemoradiation in one arm and gemcitabine before and after chemoradiation in the experimental arm. In contrast, the ESPAC-3 trial involves a randomization to chemotherapy alone without radiation based on the results of the ESPAC-1 trial. The American College of Surgeons Oncology Group (ACSOG) is evaluating a multidrug regimen incorporating radiation, infusional 5-FU, cisplatin, and interferon in a multi-institutional phase II trial based on promising results from a single-institution study. In the single-institution study from Virginia Mason, 33 patients with head of pancreas cancer received the chemoradiation regimen and had a median survival of greater than 24 months and a 2-year survival of 84%. Despite 76% of patients in this study having node-positive disease (compared to 44% in the GITSG study), the prolonged survivals constitute the best results to date for patients with locoregional pancreatic cancer.

Another area of investigation is neoadjuvant chemoradiotherapy, which has many advantages over the adjuvant approach, such as preventing the need for surgery in those who progress and potentially increasing the likelihood of achieving a curative resection. However, neoadjuvant therapy rarely converts patients from unresectable to resectable disease states, and a prospective randomized trial comparing neoadjuvant to adjuvant therapy has yet to be performed. In conclusion, adjuvant therapy should be offered to all patients post-pancreatic resection. Future studies aim to clarify the optimal type and schedule of adjuvant therapy.

The patient presented is presently receiving 5-FU–based chemoradiation.

Clinical Pearls

1. In suitable patients, surgery is the treatment of choice for resectable pancreatic cancer.

2. Morbidity from pancreatic cancer surgery is dependent on surgical expertise.

3. Adjuvant therapy should be offered to all suitable patients post-Whipple surgery. Adjuvant chemoradiation may improve the median and overall survival.

4. Neoadjuvant therapy may be useful to select outpatients not suitable for surgery or for patients with borderline resectability. It has not yet been shown to be superior to adjuvant therapy and rarely converts patients from truly unresectable to resectable disease states.

REFERENCES

1. Neoptolemos JP, Stocken DD, Friess H, et al: A randomized trial of chemoradiotherapy and chemotherapy after resection of pancreatic cancer. N Engl J Med 350:1200-1210, 2004.
2. Neoptolemos JP, Dunn JA, Stocken DD, et al: Adjuvant chemoradiotherapy and chemotherapy in resectable pancreatic cancer: A randomized controlled trial. Lancet 358:1576-1585, 2001.
3. Nukui Y, Picozzi J, Traverso LW: Interferon-based adjuvant chemoradiation therapy improves survival after pancreaticoduodenectomy for pancreatic adenocarcinoma. Am J Surg 179:367-371, 2000.
4. Klinkenbijl JH, Jeekel J, Sahmoud T, et al: Adjuvant radiotherapy and 5-fluorouracil after curative resection of cancer of the pancreas and periampullary region. Phase III trial of the EORTC Gastrointestinal Tract Cancer Cooperative Group. Ann Surg 230:776–784, 1999.
5. Bakkevold KE, Aresjo B, Dahl O, Kambestad B: Adjuvant combination chemotherapy (AMF) following radical resection of carcinoma of the pancreas and papilla of Vater-results of a controlled, prospective, randomized multicentre study. Eur J Cancer 29A:698-703, 1993.
6. Gastrointestinal Tumor Study Group: Further evidence of effective adjuvant combined radiation and chemotherapy following curative resection of pancreatic cancer. Cancer 59:2006-2010, 1987.
7. Kalser MH, Ellenberg SS: Pancreatic cancer. Adjuvant combined radiation and chemotherapy following curative resection. Arch Surg 12:899-903, 1985.

PATIENT 41

A 72-year-old woman with multiple liver metastases and diarrhea

A 72-year-old woman presents to her primary care physician with a 3-month history of nausea, abdominal cramping, and increasing diarrhea. A CT scan of the abdomen and pelvis demonstrates multiple bilateral liver lesions measuring up to 4 cm in diameter. The pancreas is noted to be somewhat "full" but without a distinct mass. There is no significant lymphadenopathy. A colonoscopy is performed, which is normal.

Past medical history is significant for Stage 0 Chronic Lymphocytic Leukemia (CLL), type II diabetes mellitus. Glucose control had been excellent but, recently, seems more sporadic. Several years ago the patient was diagnosed with coronary artery disease, and she is status post coronary artery bypass graft (CABG) surgery with an ejection fraction of 35%.

Physical Examination: General: well-appearing. Vital signs: stable. HEENT: anicteric, no lymphadenopathy. Chest: clear. Cardiac: regular rate and rhythm, without murmurs. Abdomen: liver edge is palpable 3 cm below right costal margin, no splenomegaly. Extremities: no peripheral edema.

Laboratory Findings: WBC 11,000/μL with 89% lymphocytes, hemoglobin and platelets: normal. Biochemical profile: total bilirubin and transaminases: normal. Alkaline phosphatase mildly elevated at 135 U/L.

Questions: What diagnostic tests, other than biopsy, can be performed to confirm the diagnosis? What are options for management of this patient?

Answers: In addition to biopsy, an elevated urinary 5-HIAA would confirm the diagnosis of metastatic carcinoid tumor. Treatment with octreotide is indicated.

Discussion: The presence of diffuse liver metastases in association with normal liver function tests is highly suggestive of metastatic carcinoid tumor. Diarrhea is consistent with carcinoid syndrome. An elevated urinary 5-HIAA has a sensitivity of approximately 75% and specificity of greater than 90% in diagnosing carcinoid syndrome. Limitations of this test include false positives with certain medications (phenobarbital, warfarin) and low levels in some foregut carcinoids (bronchial and stomach). In addition, an indium-111 octreotide scan can be helpful in localizing the tumor. Among patients with carcinoid syndrome, the sensitivity is reported to be as high as 90%. A liver biopsy will confirm the diagnosis in this patient.

Carcinoid tumors are low-grade neuroendocrine cancers typically described as small, regular cells with rounded blue nuclei. They arise most commonly from the lungs, gastrointestinal tract, or pancreas and are classified according to their embryological origin: foregut, midgut, and hindgut. The term *carcinoid* implies generally that the tumor is a well-differentiated, indolent tumor with little mitotic activity. Tumors that arise from the *midgut* (jejunum, ileum, appendix, and ascending colon) release typically serotonin and prostaglandins and produce the classic carcinoid syndrome. However, tumors arising from the *hindgut* or rectum do *not* release secretory products and therefore are not associated with carcinoid syndrome. Tumors arising from the *foregut* (lung, duodenum, pancreas, and bronchus) release typically serotonin and histamine and are associated with an atypical carcinoid syndrome characterized by hives. This patient had an elevated urinary 5-HIAA level and a biopsy that was consistent with a low-grade neuroendocrine tumor, metastatic carcinoid. She also had an octreotide scan that demonstrated multiple lesions in the liver and possible uptake near the hepatic flexure of the colon.

Foregut and midgut carcinoid tumors can mediate a variety of humoral factors that lead to the classic symptoms of carcinoid syndrome, such as flushing, diarrhea, and abdominal pain. Most of these mediators are metabolized by the liver, so carcinoid syndrome is seen typically in the metastatic setting only, where mediators are released into the systemic vasculature via the hepatic veins. One of the more prominent products released by carcinoid cells is serotonin. The carcinoid cell metabolizes dietary tryptophan into serotonin and releases it into the bloodstream, which stimulates intestinal secretion and motility leading to diarrhea. Serotonin is then metabolized into 5-HIAA and secreted into the urine. However, not all carcinoid tumors metabolize tryptophan. For example, tumors arising from the hindgut do not release excess serotonin and are therefore not associated with diarrhea, even in the metastatic setting.

Flushing is another prominent symptom of the carcinoid syndrome and is likely caused by release of bradykinin, although this is not clear. The typical flush of the carcinoid syndrome begins abruptly, covers the face, neck, and upper chest, and lasts for about 20 to 30 seconds. An atypical flushing can be associated with histamine release in hindgut tumors. This flushing is described as patchy, sharply demarcated areas that are pruritic and can be ameliorated with histamine antagonists. Histamine is released typically by bronchial or gastric carcinoids.

Metastatic carcinoid is typically slow-growing and very resistant to chemotherapy. The treatment approach is aimed at alleviating symptoms and improving quality of life. This can be achieved with several different approaches. The least invasive approach is treatment with the somatostatin analog, octreotide. The majority of carcinoid tumors possess high-affinity receptors for somatostatin. Octreotide acts by binding these receptors and decreasing release of serotonin and other peptides. This agent can be given as a daily subcutaneous injection or as a long-acting intramuscular injection given once per month. Complete or partial improvement in symptoms of diarrhea and flushing and a concomitant decrease in elevated 5-HIAA levels will be experienced by 60 to 70% of patients. In addition, octreotide has been shown to stabilize tumors radiographically in up to 50% of patients.

Another option is embolization or chemoembolization. Liver metastases rely on the hepatic artery for their blood supply, allowing for transarterial embolization to be effective in inducing necrosis of metastasis. This can lead to significant symptomatic improvement in greater than 50% of patients. Unfortunately, most patients will eventually progress and symptoms will recur. Embolization can last generally for 18 to 24 months. Remember to consider the morbidity of the procedure.

Other options that are less commonly employed include surgical resection (held for patients with a very limited number of hepatic metastases) and radiofrequency ablation.

In the present patient, treatment with 20 mg of long-acting octreotide given on a monthly basis was recommended. Assessment of the patient's symptoms will continue, and a CT scan of the abdomen will be obtained every 3 to 4 months. Although carcinoid is considered an indolent tumor, once patients become symptomatic with extensive hepatic metastases, the overall survival at 5 years is about 45%.

Clinical Pearls

1. An elevated urinary 5-HIAA is reported to have a sensitivity of approximately 75% and specificity of greater than 90% in diagnosing carcinoid syndrome.

2. Tumors that arise from the midgut (jejunum, ileum, appendix, and ascending colon) release typically serotonin and prostaglandins and produce the classic carcinoid syndrome.

3. Complete or partial improvement in symptoms of diarrhea and flushing and a concomitant decrease in elevated 5 -HIAA levels is experienced by 60 to 70% of patients when treated with octreotide.

REFERENCES

1. Saltz L, Trochanowski B, Buckley M, et al: Octreotide as an antineoplastic agent in the treatment of functional and nonfunctional neuroendocrine tumors. Cancer 72(1):244-248, 1993.
2. Kvols LK, Moertel CG, O'Connell MJ, et al: Treatment of the malignant carcinoid syndrome. Evaluation of a long-acting somatostatin analogue. N Engl J Med 315(11):663-666, 1986.
3. Maton PN, Camilleri M, Griffin G, et al: Role of hepatic arterial embolisation in the carcinoid syndrome. Br Med J 287(6397):932-935, 1983.

PATIENT 42

A 54-year-old woman with a large right upper lobe lung mass

A 54-year-old woman with a long history of tobacco use presents to her physician with symptoms of reflux and right-sided chest pain. She denies any additional symptoms, such as cough, shortness of breath, and weight loss.

Physical Examination: Vital signs: normal. General: well-appearing. Cardiac: regular rate and rhythm with no murmurs. Pulmonary: clear to auscultation bilaterally. Abdomen: soft, nontender, no hepatosplenomegaly. Extremities: early clubbing present.

Laboratory Findings: CBC and electrolytes: normal. Chest radiograph: large right upper lobe mass. Bronchoscopy and biopsy: consistent with non–small-cell lung cancer. CT scan of brain: normal. PET scan: uptake in lung lesion and right hilum, with slight uptake in ipsilateral hilar nodes. Mediastinoscopy: no evidence for mediastinal nodal involvement. Pulmonary function testing: FEV_1 80% predicted. CT scan of chest: large right lung lesion invading chest wall (see Figure).

Questions: What stage is the patient's non–small-cell lung cancer? Is she a surgical candidate, and, if so, should she receive any treatment prior to surgery?

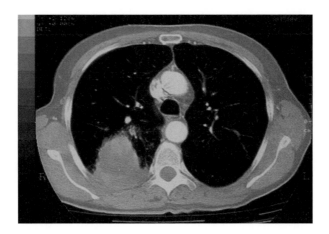

Diagnosis: This patient has stage IIIA non–small-cell lung cancer. Preoperative chemotherapy followed by surgical resection is the optimal management.

Discussion: The patient has a tumor invading the chest wall (T_3) and ipsilateral hilar lymph node involvement (N_1), without evidence of metastatic disease (M_0). By the international staging system, this corresponds to stage IIIA disease. Patients with stage IIIA non–small-cell lung cancer have regionally advanced primary cancers, with or without ipsilateral mediastinal lymph nodes. Surgical resection is possible in many of these patients, but long-term survival following surgery has been historically disappointing because of locoregional or systemic recurrence. Median survival in patients with stage IIIA disease prior to the use of preoperative chemotherapy was 12 months, with approximately 15% of patients alive at 3 years.

Preoperative *cisplatin-based combination chemotherapy* has been shown to improve the prognosis for patients with stage IIIA non–small-cell lung cancer. In a series of patients treated at Memorial Sloan Kettering, the use of preoperative mitomycin, vinblastine, and cisplatin (MVP) demonstrated major objective responses in 77% of patients, with clinical complete response on imaging studies in 10%. The overall median survival was 19 months, with 28% alive at 3 years. In several phase II trials using different cisplatin-based combinations of preoperative chemotherapy, response rates were 50 to 77%; 65 to 90% of patients had resectable tumors after chemotherapy; and median survival ranged from 13 to 32 months. A number of randomized trials have confirmed the survival benefit for this approach.

Researchers at the MD Anderson Cancer Center performed a prospective randomized study comparing the results of perioperative chemotherapy and surgery with those of surgery alone. A total of 60 patients were randomized to receive six cycles of perioperative chemotherapy (cyclophosphamide, etoposide, and cisplatin) or surgery alone. Patients treated with perioperative chemotherapy and surgery had an estimated median survival of 64 months, with 11 months for patients who received surgery alone. The 3-year estimated survival rate was 56% for the perioperative chemotherapy patients and 15% for the surgery only patients. A similar randomized trial from Europe studied the use of another preoperative cisplatin combination (mitomycin, ifosfamide, and cisplatin) for three cycles or surgery alone. This group also found an improved median survival benefit in patients treated with chemotherapy plus surgery (26 months) as compared with patients treated with surgery alone (8 months). In these studies, the best survival is observed generally among patients with a pathological complete response at the time of surgery.

The present patient was treated with three cycles of gemcitabine and cisplatin, with a good partial response to treatment. She will be restaged with a PET scan, CT chest scan, and MRI brain scan. If there is no evidence of new metastatic disease, she will be referred back to thoracic surgery for a lobectomy.

Clinical Pearls

1. Surgical resection is possible in many patients with stage IIIA non–small-cell lung cancer, but long-term survival following surgery has been historically disappointing because of locoregional or systemic recurrence.

2. In several randomized trials using different cisplatin-based combinations, preoperative chemotherapy has been shown to improve survival in patients with stage IIIA non–small-cell lung cancer.

3. In these studies, the best survival is observed generally among patients with a pathological complete response at the time of surgery.

REFERENCES

1. Kris MG, Pisters KM, Ginsberg RJ, et al: Effectiveness and toxicity of preoperative therapy in stage IIIA non–small-cell lung cancer including the Memorial Sloan-Kettering experience with induction MVP in patients with bulky mediastinal lymph node metastases (Clinical N_2). Lung Cancer 12(Suppl 1):S47-S57, 1995.
2. Rosell R, Gomez-Codina J, Camps C, et al: A randomized trial comparing preoperative chemotherapy plus surgery with surgery alone in patients with non–small-cell lung cancer. N Engl J Med 330(3):153-158, 1994.
3. Roth JA, Fossella F, Komaki R, et al: A randomized trial comparing perioperative chemotherapy and surgery with surgery alone in resectable stage IIIA non–small-cell lung cancer. J Natl Cancer Inst 86(9):673-680, 1994.

PATIENT 43

A 70-year-old woman status post right upper lobectomy

A 70-year-old woman is found on chest X-ray to have a 3-cm isolated noninvading spiculated mass in the right upper lobe of her lung. She underwent a right upper lobectomy 1 month ago, with an uncomplicated postoperative course. She presents to the oncology clinic for further management.

Physical Examination: General: well-appearing, no acute distress. Temperature 36°C, pulse 68, blood pressure 132/60 mmHg. HEENT: anicteric, no adenopathy. Cardiac: regular rate and rhythm. Chest: decreased breath sounds at the right upper lobe; otherwise, clear to auscultation. Extremities: no edema.

Laboratory Findings: Pathology from lobectomy: 1.5-cm adenocarcinoma, with 1/5 ipsilateral peribronchial lymph nodes positive for malignancy. Postoperative CT scan of chest, abdomen, and pelvis: negative for evidence of metastatic disease. Other lab data, including renal function: normal.

Questions: What is the patient's stage of disease? Is adjuvant chemotherapy indicated in this setting?

Answers: This patient's non–small-cell lung cancer is stage IIA ($T_1N_1M_0$). Platinum-based adjuvant chemotherapy may improve overall and disease-free survival.

Discussion: The primary therapy for early-stage lung cancer is surgical resection. For patients with small (< 3 cm) peripheral nodules and absence of mediastinal lymphadenopathy, lobectomy with mediastinal lymph node dissection is considered the procedure of choice. Lesser surgeries, such as wedge resection or segmentectomy, are associated with greater risks of local recurrence and cancer death.

However, removal of intrathoracic lung cancers does not necessarily result in cure, and patients may die of previously undetected micrometastatic disease. Thus, adjuvant therapy has been explored to eradicate or control micrometastatic disease.

In 1995, the Non–Small-Cell Lung Cancer Collaborative Group published a meta-analysis reporting a nonsignificant 5% absolute increase in 5-year survival with the use of adjuvant cisplatin-based chemotherapy (without radiotherapy) compared to surgery alone. In light of these nonsignificant but compelling findings, randomized controlled trials were undertaken. In early 2004, the International Adjuvant Lung Cancer Trial (IALT) Collaborative Group reported that cisplatin-based adjuvant chemotherapy significantly improved survival among patients with completely resected non–small-lung cancer (stages I–III). The absolute benefit in overall survival was 4.1% (44.5% vs 40.5%), and the benefit in 5-year disease-free survival was 5.1% (39.4% vs 34.3%).

Criticisms of this trial, which included 1867 patients from 148 centers in 33 countries, concerned the heterogeneity of the patient population, variation in chemotherapy regimens, uneven use of radiotherapy, and pooling together of multiple stages of disease. Nonetheless, this trial provided compelling evidence favoring the use of adjuvant cisplatin-based chemotherapy.

In addition to the IALT data, two phase III trials were presented at the Lung Cancer Oral Abstract Presentation Session at the American Society of Clinical Oncology (ASCO) 2004 annual meeting. Results of these two studies, JBR. 10 and CALGB 9633, further suggest a beneficial role of adjuvant chemotherapy for early stage (I-II) disease. Both trials compared the efficacy and safety of platinum-based chemotherapy in early stage patients who had surgical resection versus observation alone, over 12 to 16 weeks: cisplatin plus vinorelbine in JBR.10, and carboplatin plus paclitaxel in CALGB 9633. Both studies suggested benefit to adjuvant chemotherapy with respect to overall survival (69% for JBR.10 and 71% for CALGB 9633), and improvement in failure-free survival (30% for JBR.10 and 31% for CALGB 9633), compared to observation. These trials demonstrated an absolute survival benefit of 12 to 15% for patients receiving platinum-based adjuvant chemotherapy compared with observation alone. As a result of these data, our patient received adjuvant chemotherapy with cisplatin and vinblastine for 16 weeks.

Clinical Pearls

1. The primary therapy for early stage non–small-cell lung cancer is surgery with lobectomy.

2. Most cancers of this type (70%) recur outside of the chest and only 20% recur locally. A small number (10%) recur both locally and at distant sites.

3. Increasing evidence that platinum-based adjuvant chemotherapy may improve survival among patients with completely resected non–small-cell lung cancer.

REFERENCES

1. The International Adjuvant Lung Cancer Trial Collaborative Group. Cisplatin-based adjuvant chemotherapy in patients with completely resected non–small-cell lung cancer. N Engl J Med 350(4):351-360, 2004.
2. Ginsberg RJ: Multimodality treatment of resectable non–small-cell lung cancer. Clin Lung Cancer 1(3):94-200, 2000.
3. Mountain CF: The international system for staging lung cancer. Semin Sur Oncol 18:106-155, 2000.
4. Non–Small Cell Lung Cancer Collaborative Group. Chemotherapy in non–small-cell lung cancer: A meta-analysis using updated data on individual patients from 52 randomized trials. BMJ 311:899-909, 1995.

PATIENT 44

A 32-year-old woman with a swollen lymph node

A 32-year-old woman presents with swelling on the right side of her neck. She has no past medical history. The patient is otherwise well, has had no weight loss, and is a never-smoker.

Physical Examination: Afebrile, pulse 64, blood pressure 96/61 mmHg. General: thin. Cardiovascular: regular rate and rhythm, with no murmurs. Chest: clear to auscultation bilaterally. Abdomen: no hepatosplenomegaly. Extremities: no clubbing, cyanosis, or edema.

Laboratory Findings: CBC and electrolytes: normal. CT scan of head and neck: right supraclavicular adenopathy. Fine-needle aspiration: positive for malignant cells. Panendoscopy: no lesions. Excisional biopsy of supraclavicular node: high-grade adenocarcinoma negative for thyroglobulin and chromogranin but positive for TTF-1. PET and CT scans of lungs: 3-cm × 3.5-cm mass in right upper lobe with fluoro-2-deoxy-d-glucose (FDG) uptake in mass and mediastinum; multiple hypermetabolic foci in right supraclavicular region and right hilum (see Figure). Wedge resection of lung lesion: adenocarcinoma positive for cytokeratin and TTF-1, consistent with primary lung cancer.

Questions: What is the clinical stage of the patient's non–small-cell lung cancer? What is the optimal treatment?

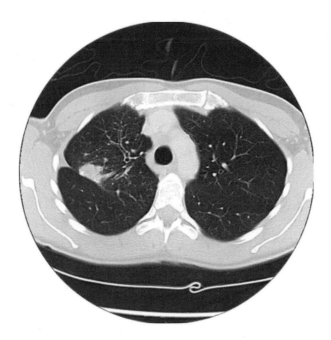

Answers: The patient has stage IIIB non–small-cell lung cancer. Concurrent chemotherapy and radiation therapy is the standard treatment approach.

Discussion: The patient has a primary tumor that is more than 3 cm in its greatest dimension (T_2), exhibits supraclavicular lymph node involvement (N_3), and is without evidence of distant metastatic disease (M_0). By the international staging system, $T_2N_3M_0$ corresponds to stage IIIB disease.

Stage IIIB disease is not considered curable by surgery because of its strong association with *micrometastatic disease.* Until the early 1990s, radiation therapy alone had been the treatment of choice for such patients, resulting in a 3-year survival of 5 to 10% and a median survival of about 10 months. Subsequently, several randomized trials demonstrated that the sequential use of cisplatin-based chemotherapy followed by radiation therapy was superior to radiation therapy alone, with improvement in median survival by 3 months on average.

In the late 1990s, studies comparing *sequential* versus *concurrent* chemoradiotherapy were reported. In one such study from Japan, median survival duration was significantly superior in patients receiving concurrent cisplatin-based chemoradiotherapy (16.5 months), as compared with those receiving sequential therapy (13.3 months). Three-year survival was 22% in the concurrent group, as compared to 15% in the sequential therapy group. Other studies performed in the United States and Europe have confirmed the improved median survival with the concurrent approach. At present, the standard of care is concurrent platinum-based chemoradiotherapy for unresectable stage III disease.

In recent years, several investigational approaches to further improve median survival in this patient group have been explored. Because distant metastases remain the major site of failure, induction chemotherapy to treat micrometastatic disease followed by concurrent chemoradiotherapy has been an approach pursued by several investigators. Others have tried the mirror approach, with concurrent chemoradiotherapy followed by consolidation with chemotherapy alone. Both approaches appear to improve median survival significantly; however, it is important to note that these studies are all phase II trials and not phase III trials. Until larger confirmatory trials are completed, these approaches should remain investigational; one such phase II study, performed by the Southwest Oncology group, evaluated consolidation *docetaxel* after concurrent cisplatin-based chemoradiotherapy. Median survival was 26 months, with a 3-year survival at an impressive 37%. The survival results from this study are the best yet for unresectable stage III patients.

The present patient was treated with cisplatin-based concurrent chemoradiotherapy and is presently receiving her third cycle of docetaxel consolidation. She has had an impressive partial response to treatment.

Clinical Pearls

1. Stage IIIB disease is not considered curable by surgery because of its strong association with micrometastatic disease.

2. Concurrent cisplatin-based chemoradiotherapy is superior to sequential therapy in patients with unresectable stage III disease.

3. Because distant metastases remain the major site of failure, promising investigational approach includes induction chemotherapy or consolidation chemotherapy following chemoradiotherapy.

REFERENCES
1. Gandara DR, Chansky K, Albain KS, et al: Consolidation docetaxel after concurrent chemoradiotherapy in stage IIIB non–small-cell lung cancer: Phase II Southwest Oncology Group Study S9504. J Clin Oncol 21(10):2004-2010, 2003.
2. Furuse K, Fukuoka M, Kawahara M, et al: Phase III study of concurrent versus sequential thoracic radiotherapy in combination with mitomycin, vindesine, and cisplatin in unresectable stage III non–small-cell lung cancer. J Clin Oncol 17(9):2692-2699, 1999.

PATIENT 45

A 23-year-old man with chest pain and a mediastinal mass

A 23-year-old man with no significant past medical history presents to the emergency department with severe right-sided chest pain. He denies any fever, cough, dyspnea, syncope, or palpitations.

Physical Examination: Temperature 36.6°C, blood pressure 127/77 mmHg, pulse 81, Karnofsky performance status 90%. HEENT: anicteric sclera, clear oropharynx. Lymph nodes: no lymphadenopathy. Heart: regular rate and rhythm, without murmurs. Chest: clear to auscultation bilaterally. Abdomen: soft, nontender, normal bowel sounds, no masses or organomegaly palpable. Extremities: no clubbing, cyanosis, or edema. Neurological: nonfocal.

Laboratory Findings: WBC 4900/μL, hemoglobin 13.3 g/dL, platelets 238,000/μL. Comprehensive metabolic panel: normal. Chest X-ray: see Figures. CT scan of chest: see Figure, next page.

Questions: What is the radiographic finding? What is the differential diagnosis for this finding?

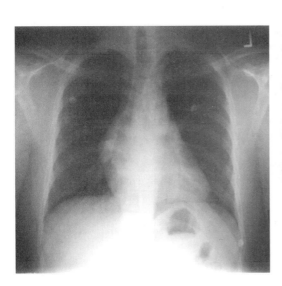 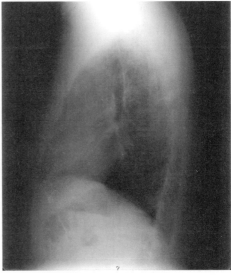

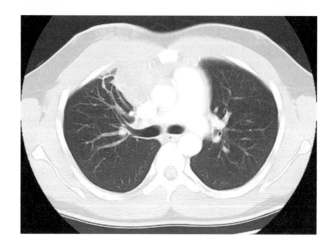

Answers: The radiographic finding is an anterior mediastinal mass. The differential diagnosis includes thymoma, lymphoma, germ cell tumor, metastatic carcinoma, sarcoma, and retrosternal goiter.

Discussion: Anterior mediastinal masses are usually malignant and have a limited differential diagnosis, which includes thymomas, lymphomas (encompassing distinct nosological entities, such as primary mediastinal lymphoma, lymphoblastic lymphoma, and diffuse large-cell lymphoma), and germ cell tumors. Thymomas are the most common of these, representing at least 30% of all anterior mediastinal masses. Other rarer tumors include sarcomas and metastatic carcinomas. A few benign entities can occur, such as retrosternal goiter and Morgagni hernias. Fine-needle aspirates are typically insufficient to differentiate the previously mentioned tumor types, and therefore core needle biopsy or surgical biopsy should be arranged. In this particular case, a core biopsy revealed malignant thymoma.

Thymomas originate from thymic epithelial cells and not from the lymphoid cells that populate the organ during their maturation. The tumor is composed of cells that have a histologically bland appearance and resemble normal thymic epithelial cells, plus variable amounts of lymphoid tissue associated with these. Thymomas can be classified into *cortical, medullary,* or *mixed type,* depending on the degree of similarity of the cells with normal cortical or medullary thymic counterparts. Medullary thymomas are believed to have a better prognosis than cortical types, but it should be noted that the behavior of a malignant thymoma is as important as histopathology to overall prognosis. A thymoma with a bland appearance that is actively invading the thymic capsule or adjacent structures, or actively metastasizing throughout the chest, has a worse prognosis than a thymoma that appears histologically more aggressive but is contained within the thymic capsule. Malignant thymomas should be distinguished from thymic carcinomas, whose cells have a malignant, nonthymic appearance under the microscope, and share an invasiveness and metastatic potential similar to non–small-cell lung cancer. Malignant thymomas are highly responsive to chemotherapy, whereas thymic carcinomas are notoriously chemoresistant.

Thymomas may present with symptoms related to invasion or compression of local structures (such as chest pain, cough, or dyspnea), and they are often associated with autoimmune phenomena. Autoimmune disorders are noted in more than two-thirds of thymomas and include neuromuscular, endocrine, and hematopoietic syndromes as well as systemic diseases (see Table). Myasthenia gravis (MG) is the most common autoimmune disorder, occurring in one of every three patients with thymoma, and, although it may affect the perioperative mortality of patients with thymoma (mostly due to myasthenic crisis), the long-term prognosis of thymoma does not appear to be influenced by the presence of MG. Resection of the thymoma does not necessarily revert the associated autoimmune syndrome, with reported remission rates varying from as high as 60% for MG to as low as zero for hypogammaglobulinemia. The patient described had no evidence of autoimmune phenomena.

Thymomas are usually staged according to the system proposed by Masaoka and colleagues, which classifies these tumors into groups with successively worse 5-year survival (from 96-50%): without capsular invasion *(stage I),* invasion into perithymic connective tissue *(stage II),* invasion into surrounding structures such as vessels (stage III), and metastatic/direct pericardial or pleural extension (stage IV). Surgery is the mainstay of treatment for stages I through III. The resection should be done through a median sternotomy with as complete a thymectomy as possible.

No adjuvant therapy is required for stage I patients following a complete surgical resection. Adjuvant radiation therapy has traditionally been given to stage III patients, and in these patients it has decreased local recurrence, but it is more controversial in stage II. Most authors do not recommend its use routinely in completely resected stage II disease, but some suggest that it should be considered strongly when fibrous adhesions to the pleura are seen during surgery. Stage IV patients are treated with chemotherapy. There are no prospective randomized trials comparing different chemotherapeutic agents, and both single-drug and combination regimens have been used with complete response rates up to 40%. Cisplatin is the most frequently used drug in combination with other agents.

More recently, a few series of stage III patients given multimodality treatment, with adjuvant cisplatin-based chemoradiation therapy, show encouraging results. Also, the use of induction (neoadjuvant) chemotherapy seems to increase the resectability of locally advanced (stage III or IV) thymoma.

The present patient, due to the size, location, and apparent extracapsular extension of the tumor, was prescribed induction chemotherapy with cisplatin and etoposide (EP) prior to being taken for surgery. He underwent sperm-banking prior to chemotherapy, in case the platinum would damage his fertility. He experienced a radiological complete response to three cycles of EP. Subsequent sternotomy and thymectomy revealed negative margins and no residual cancer (pathological complete response), and therefore no adjuvant radiation was recommended.

Autoimmune Manifestations Associated with Thymoma

Neuromuscular Disorders
    Myasthenia gravis
    Eaton-Lambert syndrome
    Stiff-person syndrome
    Polyneuropathy
    Polymyositis
Hematopoietic Disorders
    Pure red cell aplasia
    Hypogammaglobulinemia
    Pernicious anemia
    Other cytopenias
Endocrine Disorders
    Panhypopituitarism
    Hashimoto's thyroiditis
    Graves' disease
    Addison's disease
Systemic Disorders
    Systemic lupus erythematosus
    Sjögren's syndrome
    Rheumatoid arthritis
    Scleroderma
Other
    Sarcoidosis
    Nephrotic syndrome
    Hypertrophic osteoarthropathy

Data from Cameron RB, Loehrer PJ, Thomas CR: Neoplasms of the mediastinum. In DeVita VT Jr, Hellman S, Rosenberg SA (eds): Cancer: Principles & Practice of Oncology, 6th ed. Philadelphia, Lippincott, Williams & Wilkins, 2001, pp 1019-1036.

Clinical Pearls

1. Anterior mediastinal masses are almost always malignant.

2. Thymomas originate from thymic epithelial cells.

3. Thymomas are associated in 60% of cases with autoimmune phenomena, which have no major influence on prognosis. Resection of a thymoma does not necessarily resolve the associated autoimmune disease.

4. Surgery is the mainstay of treatment for localized disease.

5. Adjuvant radiation therapy is given for nonmetastatic tumors that invade through the thymic capsule into surrounding structures. Multimodality therapy, including induction chemotherapy, is also employed in these cases.

REFERENCES

1. Venuta F, Rendina EA, Longo F: Long-term outcome after multimodality treatment for stage III thymic tumors. Ann Thorac Surg 76:1866-1872; discussion 1872, 2003.
2. Johnson SB, Eng TY, Giaccone G, Thomas CR Jr: Thymoma: Update for the new millennium. Oncologist 6:239-246, 2001.
3. Cameron RB, Loehrer PJ, Thomas CRJ: Neoplasms of the mediastinum. In DeVita VTJ, Hellman S, Rosenberg SA (eds): Cancer: Principles and Practice of Oncology. Philadelphia, Lippincott Williams & Wilkins, 2000, pp 1019-1036.
4. Shin DM, Walsh GL, Komaki R, et al: A multidisciplinary approach to therapy for unresectable malignant thymoma. Ann Intern Med 129:100-104, 1998.
5. Davis RD Jr, Oldham HN Jr, Sabiston DC Jr: Primary cysts and neoplasms of the mediastinum: Recent changes in clinical presentation, methods of diagnosis, management, and results. Ann Thorac Surg 44:229-237, 1987.
6. Masaoka A, Monden Y, Nakahara K, Tanioka T: Follow-up study of thymomas with special reference to their clinical stages. Cancer 48:2485-2492, 1981.

PATIENT 46

A 49-year-old woman with cough and a lump in the left side of neck

A 49-year-old woman presents with minimally productive cough, fatigue, and a lump in the left side of neck. She has a 32-pack/year smoking history. Medical history is significant for two early-stage malignant melanomas resected from her back.

Physical Examination: General: well-appearing, no acute distress. Vital signs: temperature 35.9°C, blood pressure 103/68 mmHg, pulse 117, Karnofsky performance status 90%. HEENT: anicteric sclera, clear oropharynx. Lymph nodes: 2-cm hard left supraclavicular lymph node. Cardiovascular: tachycardic without murmurs. Chest: clear to auscultation bilaterally with scattered rhonchi. Abdomen: soft, non-tender, normal bowel sounds, no masses or organomegaly palpable. Extremities: no clubbing, cyanosis, or edema.

Laboratory Findings: CBC: hemoglobin 15 g/dL, platelets 429,000/μL; WBC 10,300/μL. Comprehensive metabolic panel: normal, including alkaline phosphatase and lactate dehydrogenase. Chest X-ray: see Figure. CT scan of chest: see Figure, next page. Histology specimen from core biopsy of supraclavicular lymphadenopathy: see Figure, next page.

Question: What is the patient's diagnosis?

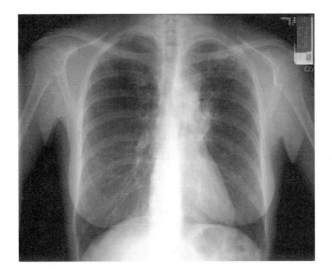

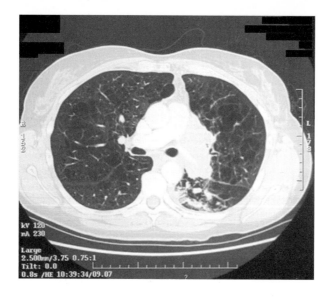

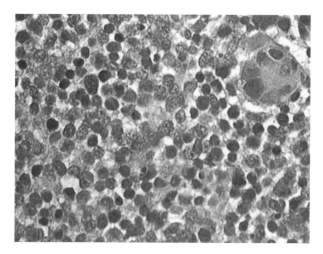

Diagnosis: Limited-stage small-cell lung cancer is the patient's diagnosis.

Discussion: This case illustrates one of the presentations of small-cell lung cancer (SCLC), which constitutes 12 to 15% of all malignant pulmonary tumors. Similar to non–small-cell lung cancer (NSCLC), there is a strong association between this tumor and smoking, with almost all cases of SCLC arising in smokers. In fact, before a diagnosis of SCLC can be made in a patient who never smoked, or never had exposure to second-hand tobacco smoke, any other potential diagnoses should be thoroughly ruled out. This patient had evidence of a left hilar mass and mediastinal lymphadenopathy (first two Figures). The classic "oat cell" component of the tumor can be seen in the third Figure.

In contrast to NSCLC, surgery plays a minor role in the treatment of SCLC, even for localized disease. This explains in part why the TNM classification is seldom used for staging of SCLC, and

instead the disease is classified into two stages: limited stage and extensive stage. *Limited stage* refers to SCLC that is confined to one hemithorax and can be included in a single radiation field. Approximately 30 to 40% of patients have limited-stage disease at presentation. *Extensive-stage* disease refers to tumors that are beyond the areas of limited disease, including contralateral hilar nodes and distant metastasis. In the patient described, the ipsilateral supraclavicular lymph node can still be covered in a single radiation field, and, therefore, her condition is consistent with limited-stage disease. To determine the feasibility of radiation and to confirm staging, consultation with a radiation oncologist is often necessary.

The distinction between limited- and extensive-stage disease is critical because treatment strategies differ. To rule out extensive-stage disease, all patients undergo a CT scan of the chest/abdomen with intravenous contrast (including the adrenal glands and entire liver). In addition, an MRI of the brain with gadolinium and a nuclear medicine test (preferably an FDG-PET scan) are mandatory. It should be noted that some FDG-PET scans do not image the long bones of the extremities, and, therefore, a bone scan may be indicated in any patient with bone pain or elevated alkaline phosphatase or lactate dehydrogenase (LDH). A CT scan of the brain with intravenous contrast is an alternative to an MRI in selected patients.

SCLC metastasizes to the bone marrow in 15 to 30% of patients, but this is usually associated with elevated LDH or alkaline phosphatase and is uncommonly the only site of metastatic disease. Therefore, a bone marrow biopsy is only recommended for patients without other evidence of extensive disease but who have an elevated LDH, alkaline phosphatase, or evidence of disturbed hematopoiesis (cytopenias). In this patient, given her normal LDH, alkaline phosphatase, and hematopoiesis, a bone marrow biopsy was not necessary before concluding that she had limited-stage disease.

Although chemotherapy is the only first-line treatment for extensive-stage disease, patients with limited-stage disease are managed with concurrent chemotherapy and radiation. Sequential chemotherapy and radiation is acceptable in elderly or poor performance-status patients with limited-stage disease. Chemotherapy plus radiation therapy, compared to chemotherapy alone, has been reported in a meta-analysis to provide a modest increase in the survival of SCLC patients. More recent trials have demonstrated that early administration of radiation with chemotherapy is beneficial, hence, the predilection to treat with concurrent chemotherapy and radiation and to begin radiation during the first or second cycle of chemotherapy.

Chemotherapy consists of usually a combination of cisplatin with etoposide given for four to six cycles. Radiation therapy is given typically once daily with the first or second cycle of chemotherapy. When radiation therapy is given twice daily (hyperfractionated), there seems to be an improvement in survival compared to conventional radiation therapy (although once daily administration is often chosen by patients and clinicians for logistical reasons).

Because there is a high risk of recurrence in the central nervous system, *prophylactic cranial irradiation* (PCI) is recommended in all SCLC patients who experience a major response to treatment (complete response or near-complete response). A meta-analysis of survival data in SCLC patients suggests that PCI decreases the risk of brain metastases and death.

The present patient was treated with a combination of cisplatin and etoposide concomitantly with hyperfractionated radiation therapy, to be followed by PCI contingent on a good response.

Clinical Pearls

1. Newly diagnosed SCLC is classified as *limited stage* or *extensive stage,* based on whether all sites of disease can be included in a single radiation field. Ipsilateral supraclavicular lymphadenopathy is considered within the boundaries of limited-stage disease. Consultation with a radiation oncologist is often necessary to determine the feasibility of radiation and to confirm staging.

2. A bone marrow biopsy is only recommended for patients without any objective evidence of extensive disease but who have an elevated LDH, alkaline phosphatase, or cytopenia.

3. The treatment of limited-stage disease involves chemotherapy combined with radiation. In extensive-stage disease, chemotherapy alone is used.

4. Prophylactic cranial irradiation (PCI) is recommended in all SCLC patients who experience a major response to treatment.

REFERENCES

1. Takada M, Fukuoka M, Kawahara M, et al: Phase III study of concurrent versus sequential thoracic radiotherapy in combination with cisplatin and etoposide for limited-stage small-cell lung cancer: Results of the Japan Clinical Oncology Group Study 9104. J Clin Oncol 20:3054-3060, 2002.
2. Auperin A, Arriagada R, Pignon JP, et al: Prophylactic cranial irradiation for patients with small-cell lung cancer in complete remission. Prophylactic Cranial Irradiation Overview Collaborative Group. N Engl J Med 341:476-484, 1999.
3. Turrisi AT III, Kim K, Blum R, et al: Twice -daily compared with once-daily thoracic radiotherapy in limited small-cell lung cancer treated concurrently with cisplatin and etoposide. N Engl J Med 340:265-271, 1999.
4. Pignon JP, Arriagada R, Ihde DC, et al: A meta-analysis of thoracic radiotherapy for small-cell lung cancer. N Engl J Med 327:1618-1624, 1992.
5. Warde P, Payne D: Does thoracic irradiation improve survival and local control in limited-stage small-cell carcinoma of the lung? A meta-analysis. J Clin Oncol 10:890-895, 1992.

PATIENT 47

A 53-year-old man with left hip pain and diffuse lymphadenopathy

A 53-year-old man presents to his physician with 6 weeks of increasing left groin pain on ambulation. The patient also describes a 2-month history of 15-pound weight loss, despite unchanged eating habits and night sweats.

Physical Examination: General: well-appearing. Blood pressure 110/76 mmHg, temperature 36.4°C. Lymph nodes: easily palpable 2-cm left supraclavicular node, 3-cm left axillary lymph nodes. Abdomen: spleen tip palpable 3 cm below left costal margin.

Laboratory Findings: CBC: normal. Chemistry profile: normal. LDH: normal at 194. MRI scan of left hip: destructive lesion of the proximal femur and surrounding soft tissue mass (see Figure). CT scan: cervical, axillary, and supraclavicular adenopathy with splenomegaly and multiple low attenuation lesions in spleen. Biopsy of left supraclavicular node: large poly-lobulated cells staining positively for CD20, and a background of numerous CD3-positive small lymphocytes. CD15, CD30, EMA, CD10, and ALK1 stains are all negative.

Question: What type of lymphoma does the patient have?

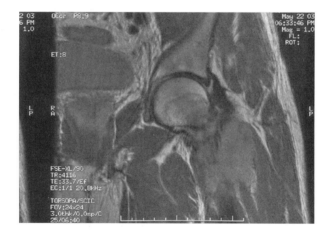

Answer: The patient has T-cell rich B-cell lymphoma.

Discussion: T-cell rich B-cell lymphoma (TCR-BCL) is a recently described histological variant of diffuse large B-cell lymphoma. It is characterized by a minor population of clonal B-cells surrounded by a majority of polyclonal T-cells. The clonal B-cell population comprises typically 10% or less of the total cellular population. Morphologically, TCR-BCL can easily be confused with other lymphomas—in particular, *lymphocyte-predominant Hodgkin's disease, classic Hodgkin's,* and *peripheral T-cell lymphoma.* Immunophenotyping studies are thus critical in establishing the diagnosis. The B-cells in the minority population stain positively for the B-cell marker CD20 but negative for CD15 and CD30, allowing a distinction from lymphocyte-rich classic Hodgkin's disease. The negative staining for anaplastic lymphoma kinase (ALK) and epithelial membrane antigen (EMA) excludes a diagnosis of anaplastic large-cell lymphoma in this patient. Lymphocyte-predominant Hodgkin's disease (LPHD) has a similar immunophenotype, with large cells staining positively for CD20 and negative for CD15 and CD30. However, the small background lymphocytes of LPHD are B-cells, whereas they are T-cells in TCR-BCL.

The clinical presentation of patients with TCR-BCL is much more akin to diffuse large B-cell lymphoma than LPHD. Patients tend to be older, presenting in their sixth or seventh decade of life, unlike LPHD for which the median age of presentation is 35 years. B symptoms (unexplained and persisting symptoms) of weight loss, night sweats, and fever are much more common in TCR-BCL and are seen infrequently in LPHD. *Extranodal involvement* is extremely rare in LPHD but is a frequent finding in TCR-BCL. *Splenomegaly* and *splenic involvement* are also much more frequently seen in TCR-BCL. Although lymphocyte-predominant Hodgkin's disease may have a similar immunophenotype, the clinical presentation of this patient is clearly much more consistent with TCR-BCL.

Staging procedures to define the anatomical extent of the disease should include a careful physical examination for lymphadenopathy and organomegaly, CT scans of the chest, abdomen, and pelvis, and a bone marrow biopsy. Central nervous system imaging with a CT scan or MRI, and evaluation of the cerebrospinal fluid, are indicated in patients with aggressive histology lymphoma involving the bone marrow. In patients who are younger than age 60, the age-adjusted *International Prognostic Index* (IPI) utilizes three factors to predict clinical outcome in adult non-Hodgkin's lymphoma: (a) the stage; (b) clinical performance status; and (c) elevated lactate dehydrogenase. The age-adjusted IPI is a simple additive score from 0 to 3 and stratifies patients into four prognostic risk categories: low risk (IPI score 0; 83% 5-year survival); low intermediate risk (IPI score 1; 69% 5-year survival); high intermediate (IPI score 2; 46% 5-year survival); and high risk (IPI score 3; 32% 5-year survival). The patient presented has low intermediate risk disease by virtue of the normal lactate dehydrogenase, good performance status, and stage IV disease.

It is of critical importance to distinguish TCR-BCL from LPHD, because non-Hodgkin's lymphoma–directed therapy with regimens, such as rituximab, cyclophosphamide, doxorubicin, vincristine, and prednisone (R-CHOP), clearly offer an advantage in disease-free survival as compared with Hodgkin's disease-related therapy. In one series of patients, disease-free survival was significantly better for non-Hodgkin's–directed chemotherapy (36%) versus Hodgkin's–directed chemotherapy (10%) at 3 years. Overall survival, however, was not statistically different due to successful salvage therapy in both groups.

The present patient was enrolled in a clinical protocol and received accelerated R-CHOP followed by ICE (ifosfamide, carboplatin, etoposide) chemotherapy. He also received intrathecal methotrexate, tolerating all treatment remarkably well. At 4 months following treatment he remains in complete clinical remission.

Clinical Pearls

1. T-cell rich B-cell lymphoma is characterized by a minor population of large clonal B-cells, surrounded by a majority of polyclonal small T-cells.

2. The B-cells in the minority population stain positively for the B-cell marker CD20 but negatively for CD15 and CD30, allowing a distinction from classic Hodgkin's disease.

3. Non-Hodgkin's lymphoma–directed therapy with regimens, such as R-CHOP, clearly offer an advantage in disease-free survival as compared with Hodgkin's disease–related therapy.

REFERENCES

1. Ripp JA, Loiue DC, Chan W, et al: T-cell rich B-cell lymphoma: Clinical distinctiveness and response to treatment in 45 patients. Leuk Lymphoma 43(8):1573-1580, 2002.
2. Rodriguez J, Pugh WC, Cabanillas F: T-cell rich B-cell lymphoma. Blood 82(5):1586-1589, 1993.

PATIENT 48

A 58-year-old woman with ductal carcinoma *in situ*

A 58-year-old postmenopausal woman presents to a medical oncologist. A mammogram performed 1 month prior revealed new microcalcifications in the upper outer quadrant of her right breast. A stereotactic core biopsy revealed ductal carcinoma *in situ* (DCIS). A lumpectomy was then performed. The patient is scheduled to start radiation therapy to the right breast. Past medical history is significant for hypercholesterolemia only. Family history is negative for malignancy. The patient had her first full-term pregnancy at age 25 and is G2P2. Menarche occurred at age 12, and menopause occurred at age 51. She has never taken oral contraceptives or hormone replacement therapy. Social history and review of systems are unremarkable.

Physical Examination: Temperature 37°C, pulse 60, blood pressure 120/82 mmHg. General: well-nourished. HEENT: no scleral icterus; mucous membranes moist; no adenopathy. Cardiovascular: regular rate and rhythm, without murmurs. Chest: clear to auscultation, status post right lumpectomy with healed scar, no breast masses. Abdomen: soft, nontender, no organomegaly, or masses. Extremities: no axillary adenopathy, no edema, or calf tenderness.

Laboratory Findings: Hemoglobin 14.2 g/dL, WBC 7000/μL, platelets 236,000/μl. Biochemistry profile: normal. Liver function tests: normal. Chest radiograph: normal. Pathology: intermediate nuclear grade DCIS of the papillary type identified in four of eight slides, marked comedonecrosis present, no invasion noted, margins uninvolved.

Questions: Besides the scheduled radiation therapy, is further therapy indicated? If so, what type of therapy and in what way can it benefit the patient?

Answers: In addition to the lumpectomy and planned radiation, this patient should consider taking tamoxifen for 5 years. Although not a necessary part of the treatment for DCIS, tamoxifen can further decrease her risk of developing recurrent breast cancer in the involved breast and can also decrease her risk of developing a new contralateral primary breast cancer. Tamoxifen will not, however, improve her overall survival and carries potential side effects, factors she will need to consider in making her treatment choice.

Discussion: Ductal carcinoma *in situ* is a non-invasive form of breast cancer. As was the case with this patient, DCIS presents most frequently as asymptomatic microcalcifications identified on mammography. The incidence of DCIS has markedly increased since the advent of screening mammography. Because most women with DCIS do not have palpable breast masses, diagnosis usually involves an image-guided core needle biopsy.

Once a diagnosis of DCIS has been made, surgical excision is required. Although outcomes for mastectomy and breast-conserving therapy for DCIS have not been compared directly, findings of equal survival with either approach for invasive breast cancer have prompted surgeons to regard breast-conserving therapy as the preferred treatment for DCIS. Breast-conserving therapy comprises lumpectomy followed by radiation. Lumpectomy is performed usually with the guidance of a wire placed into the microcalcifications preoperatively. Mastectomy is only recommended in the setting of diffuse, multifocal DCIS or if surgical margins after lumpectomy are positive, despite attempts at reexcision.

After lumpectomy, women with DCIS are at risk for developing recurrent breast cancer in the affected breast and new primary breast cancers in the contralateral breast. Radiation therapy can decrease the first of these risks. *The National Surgical Adjuvant Breast and Bowel Project* (NSABP) *B-17* trial demonstrated that radiation therapy after lumpectomy for DCIS decreases the 5-year cumulative incidences of invasive and non-invasive breast cancers in the ipsilateral breast from 10.5% and 10.4 to 2.9% and 7.5%, respectively. Despite reducing the risk of ipsilateral breast tumor recurrences, radiation for DCIS does not impact survival.

In addition to undergoing lumpectomy and radiation therapy, women with DCIS can benefit from tamoxifen, a selective estrogen receptor modulator that has antagonistic effects on breast tissue. Although not a mandatory part of therapy for DCIS, the role for tamoxifen is based on the results of two large, randomized, controlled trials. The NSABP B-24 trial demonstrated that the administration of tamoxifen for 5 years after lumpectomy and radiation for DCIS reduces the 5-year cumulative incidence of breast cancer-related events (defined as recurrent breast cancer in the ipsilateral breast, the development of new primary breast cancer in the contralateral breast, or the development of regional/distant breast cancer metastases) from 13.4 to 8.2%. Of note, the reduction of ipsilateral breast tumor recurrence seen in this study is marked especially in women under age 50, women whose surgical margins are positive, women whose DCIS has comedonecrosis, and women who present with palpable breast masses—all of whom have especially high risk of ipsilateral breast tumor recurrence. In a related chemoprevention trial, NSABP P-1, researchers demonstrated that in women at high risk for breast cancer, tamoxifen reduces the incidence of invasive breast cancer by 49% and the incidence of noninvasive breast cancer by 50%. Since the incidence of breast cancer-related events observed after lumpectomy and radiation for DCIS in the B-24 trial is higher than that observed for some of the high-risk groups for whom tamoxifen therapy is advocated based on the results of the P-1 trial, many oncologists use the results of the B-24 and P-1 trials as the basis for considering tamoxifen therapy after lumpectomy and radiation for DCIS.

It should be noted, however, that neither the P-1 nor the B-24 trials demonstrate a survival advantage for tamoxifen therapy. In addition, both studies note adverse events associated with tamoxifen therapy. These include an increased risk of early-stage endometrial cancer and increased risks of deep vein thrombosis, pulmonary embolism, and cataracts. In addition, the incidence of strokes is insignificantly increased in women who take tamoxifen. Furthermore, symptoms, such as hot flashes and vaginal discharge, occur more frequently in women taking tamoxifen. Many of these adverse events occur more frequently in women over age 50.

After undergoing lumpectomy and radiation therapy for DCIS, all women (regardless of whether they choose to take tamoxifen for 5 years) should be followed clinically for evidence of local recurrence and the development of new primary breast cancers. Follow-up involves usually mammography each year and a physician visit every 6 months for 5 years and annually thereafter.

The present patient elected to take tamoxifen. She is tolerating this therapy without complication.

Clinical Pearls

1. Ductal carcinoma *in situ* (DCIS) presents most frequently with microcalcifications found upon screening mammography.

2. The primary treatment for DCIS is breast-conserving therapy, which involves lumpectomy followed by radiation. The use of radiation after lumpectomy for DCIS decreases the risk of developing recurrent breast cancer in the involved breast.

3. Although not a necessary part of the treatment for DCIS, tamoxifen therapy for 5 years after lumpectomy and radiation can further decrease the risk of developing recurrent breast cancer in the involved breast and can decrease the risk of developing new primary breast cancer in the contralateral breast.

4. Tamoxifen therapy is associated with potentially significant adverse events, including increased risks of early-stage endometrial cancer, deep vein thrombosis, pulmonary embolism, cataracts, and possibly stroke.

REFERENCES

1. Morrow M, Strom ER, Bassett LW, et al: Standard for the management of ductal carcinoma *in situ* of the breast (DCIS). CA Cancer J Clin 52(5):256-276, 2002.
2. Fisher B, Dignam J, Wolmark N, et al: Tamoxifen in treatment of intraductal breast cancer: National Surgical Adjuvant Breast and Bowel Project B-24 randomized controlled trial. Lancet 353(9169):1993-2000, 1999.
3. Fisher B, Costantino JP, Wickerham DL, et al: Tamoxifen for prevention of breast cancer: Report of the National Surgical Adjuvant Breast and Bowel Project P-1 Study. J Natl Cancer Inst 90(18):1371-1388, 1998.
4. Fisher B, Dignam J, Wolmark N, et al: Lumpectomy and radiation therapy for the treatment of intraductal breast cancer: Findings from the National Surgical Adjuvant Breast and Bowel Project B-17. J Clin Oncol 16(2):441-452, 1998.
5. Ernster VL, Barclay J, Kerlikowske K, et al: Incidence of and treatment for ductal carcinoma in situ of the breast. JAMA 275(12):913-918, 1996.
6. Fisher B, Costantino J, Redmond C, et al: Lumpectomy compared with lumpectomy and radiation therapy for the treatment of intraductal breast cancer. N Engl J Med 328(22):1581-1586, 1993.

PATIENT 49

A 61-year-old woman with hepatomegaly and lower extremity edema

A 61-year-old woman, without significant past medical history, presents to her primary care physician with intermittent lower extremity edema of 3-month duration. The initial exam was remarkable for hepatomegaly and trace lower extremity edema. Review of systems was otherwise unremarkable. A diagnostic procedure was performed at the referring institution.

Physical Examination: Temperature 36.6°C, pulse 96, blood pressure 120/60 mmHg. HEENT: sclerae anicteric, no macroglossia. Lymph nodes: no cervical, supraclavicular, axillary, or inguinal lymphadenopathy. Cardiovascular: regular rate and rhythm, no S3, no murmurs, no jugular venous distension (JVD). Chest: clear throughout. Abdomen: hepatomegaly 4 cm below the right costal margin at the mid-clavicular line, mild splenomegaly. Extremities: 2-positive bilateral lower extremity edema.

Laboratory Findings: Hemoglobin 12 g/dL, WBC 4600/µL, platelets 160,000/µL, total cholesterol 448 mg/dL, albumin 3.1 g/dL, creatinine 1.9 mg/dL. Twenty-four-hour urine collection: total protein 4800 mg, creatinine clearance 21 mL/min. Serum immunofixation: IgG-λ monoclonal protein 0.7 mg/dL. Bone marrow biopsy: increased number of λ-restricted plasma cells. Abdominal ultrasound: mild, fatty infiltration of somewhat enlarged liver. Skeletal survey: unremarkable. Echocardiogram and electrocardiogram: normal.

Question: What plasma cell disorders should be considered in the patient?

Answer: In a patient with monoclonal gammopathy and nephrotic range proteinuria, possible diagnoses include multiple myeloma, monoclonal gammopathy of uncertain significance, and primary systemic amyloidosis. This patient had an abdominal fat pad biopsy, which, after staining with Congo red, showed green birefringence under polarized light, confirming the diagnosis of primary systemic amyloidosis.

Discussion: Primary systemic amyloidosis is a disorder of protein conformation and a plasma cell dyscrasia. An abnormal clone of plasma cells produces an excess of immunoglobulin light chains which, along with other proteins, form amyloid fibrils. These amyloid fibrils can deposit in a variety of organs. Amyloidosis presents with a variety of syndromes reflecting the organs involved. The most frequent presentations are proteinuria (> 500 mg/day albuminuria) and dyspnea on exertion, reflecting amyloid involvement of the kidneys or heart. Other relatively common presentations include hepatomegaly, carpal tunnel syndrome, polyneuropathy, and orthostatic hypotension. Although the diagnosis can be made by biopsy of an affected organ, this is often not necessary. Congo red staining of abdominal fat pad aspirate can have a sensitivity of 85%. The diagnosis can also be made from rectal biopsy.

Initial evaluation of the patient with amyloidosis should include assessment of function of the major organ systems that are affected by the disease. This evaluation begins with a complete medical history and physical exam. The physical exam includes an assessment of orthostatic vital signs, liver span, and cardiac function, and an assessment of the tongue. Laboratory evaluation includes CBC, measurement of serum creatinine, 24-hour urine total protein, immunofixation and electrophoresis of serum and urine, and measurement of serum-free light chains. Cardiac testing includes measurement of B-type natriuretic peptide and troponin, an electrocardiogram, and an echocardiogram. Testing should also include measurement of fecal occult blood to screen for gastrointestinal tract involvement.

The prognosis for patients with amyloidosis is heavily dependent on the organ involvement and can be affected by treatment. Although patients who present with cardiac involvement have a median survival of 4 months, the median overall survival of patients treated with colchicine alone is on the order of 8 months from the time of diagnosis. With the addition of intermittent treatment with melphalan and prednisone, median survival can be prolonged significantly to 18 months. However, there is a relatively limited response rate of approximately 30%. More recently, investigations have centered on the use of early treatment with high-dose intravenous melphalan and autologous hematopoietic stem cell transplant. In selected populations, approximately two-thirds of patients show an improvement in organ function.

Measurement of response to treatment is difficult. Although production of new amyloid may be disrupted by treatment, the resorption of amyloid fibrils is a slow process and may require months.

The present patient was treated with upfront autologous stem cell transplantation as part of a clinical trial. Her dose of melphalan was adjusted based on a variety of risk factors, including her age, measured creatinine clearance, and organ involvement.

Clinical Pearls

1. In a patient with monoclonal gammopathy and symptoms out of proportion to known medical problems, suspect systemic amyloidosis.

2. Assessment of cardiac involvement in primary systemic amyloidosis is possible by measuring serum levels of brain natriuretic peptide and troponin and obtaining an electrocardiogram and echocardiogram.

3. Measurement of serum-free light chains can be helpful in quantitating response to treatment.

REFERENCES

1. Comenzo RL, Gertz MA: Autologous stem cell transplantation for primary systemic amyloidosis. Blood 99(12):4276-4282, 2002.
2. Kyle RA, Gertz MA, Greipp PR, et al: A trial of three regimens for primary amyloidosis: Colchicine alone, melphalan and prednisone, and melphalan, prednisone, and colchicine. N Engl J Med 336:1202-1207, 1997.

PATIENT 50

A 52-year-old woman with abdominal pain and jaundice

A 52-year-old woman presents to her internist complaining of intermittent abdominal pain of 2-month duration. The pain is in the right upper quadrant and radiates to the back. Over the preceding week she has become visibly jaundiced. Her past medical history is significant for *Helicobacter pylori* infection, previously treated with antibiotics and proton pump inhibitor. She has no history of alcohol or illicit substance abuse.

Physical Examination: General: icteric. Vital signs: stable. Lymph nodes: no palpable adenopathy. Cardiovascular: regular rate and rhythm. Pulmonary: clear to auscultation bilaterally. Abdomen: soft, nontender, no masses, or hepatosplenomegaly. Extremities: no clubbing, cyanosis, or edema.

Laboratory Findings: CBC: normal. Total bilirubin 5.8, γ-glutamyl transferase (GGT) 74, alkaline phosphatase 450. Abdominal ultrasound: marked dilatation of intrahepatic biliary ducts and porta hepatis mass with portal adenopathy. CT scan: multilobed mass in porta hepatis and adenopathy encasing hepatic artery with narrowing of portal vein; gastrohepatic, para-aortic, and portacaval adenopathy also seen.

Course: Endoscopic retrograde cholangiopancreatography (ERCP) and stenting are successfully performed (see Figure; biliary dilatation is now mild to moderate). Cytology from biliary duct brushings return positive for adenocarcinoma. After review by a hepatobiliary surgeon, the patient is deemed to have unresectable disease.

Questions: What is the likely diagnosis? What are the therapeutic options for this patient?

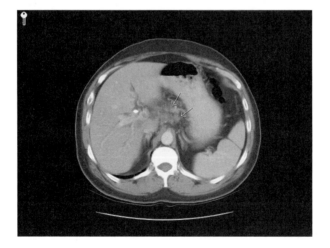

Answers: Cholangiocarcinoma is the likely diagnosis. Surgical resection, if possible, is the only curative option. Chemoradiotherapy or systemic chemotherapy with 5-FU or gemcitabine provides palliative benefit.

Discussion: Approximately 7500 new cases of biliary tract cancer are diagnosed each year. About 5000 of these are gall bladder cancers, and between 2000 and 3000 are bile-duct cancers. The term *cholangiocarcinoma* (CC) was first used to designate primary tumors of the intrahepatic bile ducts, but it is now used to include intrahepatic, perihilar (Klatskin tumors), and distal extrahepatic tumors of the bile ducts. About 60% of all cases of CC are perihilar tumors, about 20% are distal extrahepatic tumors, and the remainder are intrahepatic. CC is slightly more common in men.

Both intrahepatic and extrahepatic CCs are known complications of inflammatory conditions, such as primary sclerosing cholangitis (PSC) and ulcerative colitis. The lifetime risk of developing CC in patients with PSC is 10 to 15%. Other conditions associated with CC include bile-duct abnormalities, such as Caroli's disease (cystic dilatation of intrahepatic ducts), biliary papillomatosis, choledochal cysts, and bile duct adenomas. In southeast Asia, parasitic infestations from *Opisthorchis viverrini* and *Opisthorchis sinensis* are associated with a 25- to 50-fold increase in the risk of CC.

Extrahepatic CC presents usually with symptoms and signs of bile-duct obstruction, such as jaundice, pale stools, dark urine, and pruritus. Intrahepatic CC may present as a mass or with vague symptoms, such as pain, anorexia, weight loss, night sweats, and malaise. Laboratory investigations demonstrate typically a cholestatic picture, with mild to moderate increases in serum levels of alkaline phosphatase, bilirubin, and GGT. A CA19-9 level greater than 100 U/mL is highly suggestive of malignancy. Imaging studies begin typically with an abdominal ultrasound. This may show biliary ductal dilatation or a mass in the case of intrahepatic CC. CT scanning easily detects mass lesions and dilated biliary ducts and can be used to direct CT-guided biopsies. CT may also show regional lymphadenopathy. Magnetic resonance cholangiopancreatography allows excellent visualization of biliary anatomy and vascular structures and is becoming the imaging study of choice in patients with CC. Endoscopic ultrasound scan and PET scanning are also increasingly employed for staging patients. ERCP provides additional anatomical information and may be used to obtain a tissue diagnosis. Cytology brushings have a low yield in making a diagnosis (30%). However, in combination with biopsy, the yield can be improved to 70%.

The staging of cancers of the extrahepatic biliary tract is based on the TNM classification. In stage I, tumor invasion is limited to the biliary tree mucosa, muscle layer, or ampulla. In stage II, local invasion into liver, gallbladder, pancreas, or unilateral branches of portal vein or hepatic artery is seen. In stage III, there are metastases into regional and hepatoduodenal lymph nodes or direct invasion of tumor in the main portal vein, bilateral branches, or common hepatic artery. Stage IV cancer is characterized by extensive liver involvement, or distant metastases. Intrahepatic cancers are classified as per primary hepatic tumors.

Surgical excision is the only curative option and is possible in 30 to 60% of patients. The major step forward in surgical management of bile duct cancers was the recognition that liver resection as well as bile duct resection and reconstruction should be undertaken as an integral step in optimizing the efficacy of surgery. The goals of surgery are to excise all detectable disease and to restore biliary drainage. Laparoscopic evaluation should be considered before a formal laparotomy is performed, to identify any peritoneal metastases or noncontiguous liver metastases, thus avoiding an unnecessary laparotomy. Intrahepatic CC is treated generally by resection of the involved segments of liver and is associated with an 18- to 30-month median survival. Intrahepatic CC is increasingly recognized as a stand-alone diagnosis; however, it still requires a thorough GI workup and is often a diagnosis of exclusion, that is, after a primary site in the bowel or upper GI tract has been ruled out. Extrahepatic perihilar CC requires an en bloc resection of extrahepatic bile ducts, gall bladder, and regional lymph nodes and a Roux-en-Y hepaticojejunostomy. Partial hepatic resection may be required for tumors occluding the common hepatic duct or multicentric tumors. In distal extrahepatic tumors and cancers of the ampulla of Vater, pancreaticoduodenectomy is the therapy of choice.

The median survival for patients with perihilar and distal extrahepatic CC is 12 to 24 months, with 5-year survival rates of 15 to 25%. The 5-year survival rates for patients with periampullary cancers is considerably better (50-60%), because these patients present with symptoms and signs at an earlier stage of disease. The factors most influential in predicting recurrence include a positive surgical margin, node-positive disease, and vascular involvement by tumor. Liver transplantation has been reported to result in long-term survival in highly selected patients; however, this remains an experimental approach.

The role of adjuvant radiation therapy or chemotherapy after successful surgical resection remains controversial. Many clinicians advocate postoperative irradiation with or without systemic chemotherapy. External beam radiation and boost doses with intraluminal brachytherapy are used. The results of studies employing these approaches have been mixed; thus, in clinical practice, adjuvant therapy is generally offered to only patients with a positive margin or in the setting of lymph node metastases.

In unresectable disease, palliative treatment should be first directed at relieving biliary obstruction. This may be achieved by Roux-en-Y choledochojejunostomy or with percutaneous or endoscopically placed stents. Palliative antitumor treatments, such as chemotherapy, radiotherapy, or both, should be considered, but there is little evidence that these modalities prolong survival significantly. At present, 5-FU and cisplatin or 5-FU and gemcitabine have been shown to result in partial responses in 20 to 40% of patients. Other agents with modest activity include irinotecan, oxaliplatin, docetaxel, and mitomycin.

The present patient was not deemed a surgical candidate by virtue of the degree of vascular involvement and distant nodal involvement. She is presently receiving chemotherapy with gemcitabine and oxaliplatin.

Clinical Pearls

1. The term cholangiocarcinoma (CC) was first used to designate primary tumors of the intrahepatic bile ducts, but it is now used to include intrahepatic, perihilar (Klatskin tumors), and distal extrahepatic tumors of the bile ducts.

2. Both intrahepatic and extrahepatic CCs are known complications of inflammatory conditions, such as primary sclerosing cholangitis (PSC) and ulcerative colitis. The lifetime risk of developing CC in patients with PSC is 10 to 15%.

3. Magnetic resonance cholangiopancreatography allows excellent visualization of biliary anatomy and vascular structures and is becoming the imaging study of choice in patients with CC.

4. Surgical excision is the only curative option and is possible in 30 to 60% of patients.

5. The factors most influential in predicting recurrence after surgery include a positive surgical margin, node-positive disease, and vascular involvement by tumor.

REFERENCES

1. Fong Y, Kemeny N, Lawrence TS: Cancers of the liver and biliary tree. In Devita VT, Hellman S, Rosenberg SE (eds): Cancer: Principles and Practice of Oncology, 6th ed. Philadelphia, Lippincott, Williams & Wilkins, 2001, pp 1162-1202.
2. De Groen PC, Gores GJ, LaRusso NF, et al: Biliary tract cancers. N Engl J Med 341(18):1368-1378, 1999.

PATIENT 51

A 48-year-old woman with stage II breast cancer

A 48-year-old premenopausal woman presents to a medical oncologist after undergoing a mastectomy. Two months ago, she palpated a mass in her left breast. Her primary physician ordered a mammogram, which revealed a spiculated mass in the upper outer quadrant of the left breast. A core biopsy revealed malignancy. She then underwent a left modified radical mastectomy. Her past medical history is remarkable only for sinusitis. Family history includes a sister who died from breast cancer at the age of 43. Review of systems is unremarkable.

Physical Examination: Temperature 36.6°C, pulse 66, blood pressure 136/68 mmHg. General: well-nourished. HEENT: no scleral icterus, mucous membranes moist. Neck: no adenopathy. Cardiovascular: regular rate and rhythm, without murmurs. Chest: clear to auscultation, status post left mastectomy with healed scar, right breast without masses. Abdomen: soft, nontender, no organomegaly or masses. Extremities: no axillary adenopathy, no edema, or calf tenderness.

Laboratory Findings: Hemoglobin 12.2 g/dL, WBC 5000/μL, platelets 366,000/μL. Biochemistry profile: normal. Liver function tests: normal. Chest radiograph: normal. CT scan of chest, abdomen, and pelvis: no evidence of metastatic disease. Bone scan: no evidence of bone metastases. MUGA scan: normal ejection fraction. Pathology: 3-cm invasive ductal carcinoma, poorly differentiated, lymphovascular invasion present, estrogen and progesterone receptor negative, margins negative, HER2neu amplified, 4 of 17 axillary lymph nodes positive for metastatic breast cancer.

Questions: What types of additional therapy are indicated? How will they benefit the patient?

Answers: The patient should receive adjuvant chemotherapy and post-mastectomy radiation. Adjuvant chemotherapy has been shown to decrease breast cancer recurrence rates and to improve overall survival in early-stage breast cancer patients. Post-mastectomy radiation will further decrease her risk of locoregional recurrence and may improve her disease-free and overall survival. Adjuvant hormonal therapy is *not* indicated in women with hormone-receptor–negative breast cancer.

Discussion: The patient has stage II breast cancer. She has already undergone a mastectomy and now presents for recommendations regarding additional therapy. Important factors to consider in making treatment recommendations for this patient include her tumor size, lymph node status, and hormone receptor status.

In 2000, the National Institutes of Health convened a consensus conference to develop guidelines for the administration of adjuvant therapy for early-stage breast cancer. According to these guidelines, cytotoxic chemotherapy is recommended for women with positive axillary lymph nodes and for women with tumors larger than 1 cm. Adjuvant hormonal therapy is recommended for all patients with hormone-receptor–positive breast cancers.

Based on these guidelines, this patient should receive adjuvant cytotoxic chemotherapy. Data do not support the use of adjuvant hormonal therapy for hormone-receptor–negative patients because the effects in this group are small. The rationale for the administration of systemic adjuvant cytotoxic chemotherapy for patients with early-stage breast cancer is that, despite having undergone surgical removal of all known breast cancer, patients may still harbor microscopic metastases that could, ultimately, develop into clinically evident recurrence and lead to death.

The recommendation for chemotherapy in patients with node-positive breast cancer is supported by the findings of a meta-analysis combining the results of 47 trials of adjuvant cytotoxic chemotherapy regimens for breast cancer. The results of this meta-analysis indicate both a decrease in the risk of recurrence and a survival benefit with the administration of adjuvant cytotoxic chemotherapy for early-stage breast cancer patients. For women under age 50, chemotherapy decreases the risk of recurrence by 35% and improves overall survival by 27%. For women ages 50 to 69, chemotherapy decreases the risk of recurrence by 20% and improves overall survival by 11%. There are not enough data in the overview available for women over age 70 to describe their benefits from adjuvant chemotherapy. Although this meta-analysis demonstrates benefit from adjuvant cytotoxic chemotherapy for all patients with early-stage breast cancer, the absolute benefit of chemotherapy is noted to be greatest among young patients with positive lymph nodes, such as this patient.

There is no single adjuvant chemotherapy regimen that represents the standard of care for early-stage breast cancer patients; however, regimens containing an anthracycline appear to be slightly more effective in terms of recurrence prevention and may improve survival in comparison with non-anthracycline containing regimens. Furthermore, the addition of a taxane to the chemotherapy regimen for women with positive lymph nodes has recently been shown to further decrease recurrence and improve overall survival.

How chemotherapy is given may also be important. Retrospective studies consistently suggest that maintenance of planned dose intensity correlates with outcomes. Prospectively, it has recently been shown that increasing dose density (the dose administered per unit of time) improves disease-free and overall survival using standard doses of doxorubicin, cyclophosphamide, and paclitaxel. In this randomized trial, the chemotherapy was given to lymph node-positive breast cancer patients every 14 days with growth-factor support or every 21 days (standard) without growth factor support, and the former schedule was superior.

In addition to adjuvant chemotherapy, the patient should also receive post-mastectomy radiation therapy. The American Society of Clinical Oncology recently released clinical practice guidelines regarding the use of post-mastectomy radiation therapy. According to these guidelines, women with four or more positive axillary lymph nodes and women with tumors larger than 5 cm, or with locally advanced operable tumors, should receive post-mastectomy radiation therapy. These recommendations are based on the fact that such therapy reduces the risk of locoregional recurrence and that it may reduce the risk of distant recurrence and, ultimately, death.

Clinical Pearls

1. The rationale for the administration of systemic adjuvant therapy for patients with early-stage breast cancer is that, despite having undergone surgical removal of all known breast cancer, patients may still harbor microscopic metastases that could, ultimately, develop into clinically evident recurrence and lead to death.

2. Cytotoxic chemotherapy is recommended for women with positive axillary lymph nodes and for women with tumors larger than 1 cm. Cytotoxic chemotherapy decreases the risk of recurrence and improves overall survival. Benefits are particularly great in young women with positive lymph nodes.

3. There is no single standard regimen for adjuvant chemotherapy in breast cancer. Regimens containing anthracyclines and taxanes appear to offer superior benefit in node-positive disease. In addition, regimens with enhanced dose intensity offer greater benefit.

4. Data do not support the use of adjuvant hormonal therapy for hormone-receptor–negative patients.

5. Women with four or more positive axillary lymph nodes, tumors larger than 5 cm, or locally advanced operable tumors should receive post-mastectomy radiation therapy.

REFERENCES

1. Citron ML, Berry DA, Cirrincione C, et al: Randomized trial of dose-dense versus conventionally scheduled and sequential versus concurrent combination chemotherapy as postoperative adjuvant treatment of node positive primary breast cancer: First report of the intergroup trial C 9741/cancer and leukemia group B trial 9741. J Clin Oncol 21(8):1431-1439, 2003.
2. Henderson IC, Berry DA, Demetri GD, et al: Improved outcomes from adding sequential paclitaxel but not from escalating doxorubicin dose in an adjuvant chemotherapy regimen for patients with node-positive primary breast cancer. J Clin Oncol 21(6):976-983, 2003.
3. Early Breast Cancer Trialists' Collaborative Group. Polychemotherapy for early breast cancer: An overview of the randomized trials. Lancet 352(9132):930-942, 1998.
4. Recht A, Edge SB, Solin LJ, et al: Postmastectomy radiotherapy: Clinical practice guidelines of the American Society of Clinical Oncology. J Clin Oncol 19(5):1539-1569, 2001.
5. Anonymous. National Institutes of Health Consensus Development Conference Statement: Adjuvant therapy for breast cancer, November 1-3, 2000. J Natl Cancer Inst 93(13):979-989, 2001.
6. Early Breast Cancer Trialists' Collaborative Group. Tamoxifen for early breast cancer: An overview of the randomized trials. Lancet 351(9114):1451-1467, 1998.

PATIENT 52

A 59-year-old woman experiencing
abdominal discomfort on adjuvant tamoxifen

A 59-year-old woman was first diagnosed with an infiltrating ductal carcinoma of the right breast 3 years ago. The tumor was 2 cm, poorly differentiated, and estrogen- and progesterone-receptor positive. Three of 11 axillary lymph nodes removed at surgery were positive for metastatic carcinoma. HER2neu status was 3+ by immunohistochemistry. She was treated with a lumpectomy, axillary dissection, and four cycles of doxorubicin–cyclophosphamide followed by four cycles of paclitaxel. She then received breast irradiation and was started on tamoxifen. A month ago while continuing tamoxifen, she begun to complain of shortness of breath, cough, and right upper quadrant (RUQ) abdominal discomfort.

Physical Examination: General: no acute distress. Vital signs: stable. HEENT: anicteric with no pallor. Cardiac: regular rate and rhythm. Chest: clear to auscultation bilaterally. Abdomen: soft with mild RUQ tenderness and palpable liver edge 3 cm below costal edge.

Laboratory Findings: CBC: normal. Chemistry panel: normal. Chest X-ray: multiple pulmonary nodules. CT of abdomen: hepatic nodules. Liver biopsy: metastatic adenocarcinoma ER(+); HER2neu is now 2+ by immunohistochemistry.

Question: Is any additional testing required on the liver biopsy specimen to guide treatment decisions?

Answer: Fluorescence *in situ* hybridization (FISH) is required to confirm HER-2-neu status. This patient has significant symptoms related to visceral involvement with metastatic, HER-2-neu positive breast adenocarcinoma. Optimal treatment is with chemotherapy and trastuzumab.

Discussion: Approximately 30% of all breast cancers overexpress HER-2-neu, a 185-kD transmembrane glycoprotein receptor. Women with breast cancers that overexpress HER-2-neu have an aggressive form of the disease with a shortened disease-free survival and overall survival. Trastuzumab is a recombinant, humanized monoclonal antibody that is specific for the extracellular domain of HER-2. In preclinical studies, this antibody was found to inhibit tumor growth when used alone but also had synergistic effects when used in combination with a number of chemotherapy agents.

Testing for HER-2 overexpression has become a standard part of the pathological evaluation in women with metastatic breast cancer. Immunohistochemistry (IHC) and FISH are currently the primary techniques used for measuring this overexpression. IHC assays, such as the HercepTest, measure surface expression of the HER-2 receptor. Expression results are reported as 0, 1+, 2+, or 3+, with 3+ identifying tumors that overexpress HER-2, 2+ representing indeterminate HER-2 expression, and 1+ and 0 representing lack of HER-2 expression. FISH measures the copy number of the HER-2 gene and appears to be more reliable than IHC. Tumors that score 3+ on IHC are almost always positive by FISH. Similarly, tumors that score 0 or 1+ by IHC are negative by FISH 97% of the time. IHC 2+ tumors are found to be positive by FISH in approximately 20% of cases. All IHC 2+ tumors should be confirmed as having evidence of gene amplification by FISH prior to commencing trastuzumab therapy.

Many chemotherapy agents used in the treatment of metastatic breast cancer have demonstrated additive or synergistic antitumor activity with trastuzumab. These agents include paclitaxel, docetaxel, cyclophosphamide, epirubicin, etoposide, cisplatin, and vinorelbine. The pivotal trial demonstrating the superiority of a trastuzumab chemotherapy combination over chemotherapy alone was with paclitaxel. Slamon and colleagues reported results from a randomized multicenter study in which more than 400 women with HER-2 positive metastatic breast cancer were randomized to receive chemotherapy alone or chemotherapy with trastuzumab. Patients who had not received an anthracycline in the adjuvant setting were randomized to doxorubicin–cyclophosphamide with or without trastuzumab. If previously treated with anthracycline-based adjuvant therapy, patients received paclitaxel with or without trastuzumab. The addition of trastuzumab to chemotherapy resulted in a superior objective response rate (50 vs 32%, $p < 0.001$), a longer time to disease progression (7 vs 5 months, $p < 0.001$), a longer duration of response (9 vs 6 months, $p < 0.001$), and longer overall survival (25 vs 20 months, $p = 0.046$). The most significant adverse effect was cardiac dysfunction, which occurred in 27% of the group treated with anthracycline, cyclophosphamide, and trastuzumab. Cardiac dysfunction occurred in 13% of the group treated with paclitaxel and trastuzumab. Based on these results, *paclitaxel–trastuzumab* is the FDA-approved standard for HER-2 positive metastatic breast cancer. The significant cardiac toxicity with the anthracycline–trastuzumab combination currently precludes the use of such combinations in clinical practice.

Recently, a similarly designed study has reported significant clinical benefit in patients treated with *docetaxel–trastuzumab* when compared with docetaxel alone. Overall survival was improved from 18 months in the docetaxel alone group to 27 months in patients receiving docetaxel–trastuzumab. Ongoing studies are exploring the benefit of the addition of carboplatin to the taxane–trastuzumab combinations, with promising initial results. Weekly dosing of chemotherapy also appears to result in greater efficacy and less toxicity for taxane–trastuzumab combinations. Studies to determine the safety and efficacy of trastuzumab in the adjuvant setting are currently ongoing.

The present patient was treated weekly with paclitaxel and trastuzumab. She had an excellent response to treatment, with resolution of her symptoms and significant reduction in her disease burden. She is presently receiving her fifth cycle of chemotherapy.

Clinical Pearls

1. Women with breast cancers that overexpress HER-2 have an aggressive form of the disease with a shortened disease-free survival and overall survival.

2. All tumors determined to be 2+ by immunohistochemistry should be confirmed positive with FISH before commencing trastuzumab therapy.

3. Trastuzumab and taxane combination chemotherapy is a standard first-line therapy for HER-2 overexpressing metastatic breast cancer. The addition of carboplatin to trastuzumab–taxane combinations is emerging as a useful alternative treatment.

4. Cardiac toxicity currently precludes the use of anthracycline–trastuzumab combinations in clinical practice.

REFERENCES

1. Vogel CL, Franco SX: Clinical experience with trastuzumab (Herceptin). Breast J 9(6):452-462, 2003.
2. Slamon DJ, Leyland-Jones B, Shak S: Use of chemotherapy plus a monoclonal antibody against HER-2 for metastatic breast cancer that overexpresses HER-2. N Engl J Med 344(11):783-791, 2001.

PATIENT 53

A 72-year-old man with a large left upper lobe lung mass

A 72-year-old man is evaluated by his physician for left axilla pain radiating down the inner aspect of his arm, 15-pound weight loss, and a chronic cough. He gives a long history of tobacco use but has no other past medical history.

Physical Examination: General: well-appearing, thin. Vital signs: stable. HEENT: anisocoria with small left pupil. Lymph nodes: no palpable adenopathy. Cardiac: regular rate and rhythm. Chest: clear to auscultation bilaterally. Abdomen: soft, nontender, no hepatomegaly. Extremities: no cyanosis or edema; early clubbing noted.

Laboratory Findings: CBC and biochemistry profiles: normal. Chest X-ray: large left upper lobe mass. CT scan of chest: large 6 cm × 8 cm left upper lobe mass abutting apical aspect of chest wall (see Figure). MRI of brachial plexus: no displacement of plexus or infiltration of individual nerves. Surgical pathology following bronchoscopy and biopsy of mass: consistent with non–small-cell lung cancer. Mediastinoscopy: no evidence of mediastinal involvement. MRI and PET scans of brain: no evidence of distant metastatic disease.

Questions: What is the likely diagnosis? What is the optimum treatment approach for the patient?

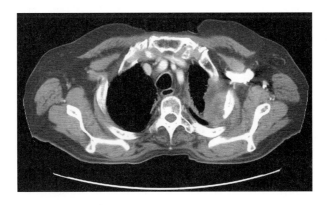

Answers: Non–small-cell lung carcinoma of the superior sulcus is the likely diagnosis. Induction chemoradiation followed by surgical resection is the standard treatment approach.

Discussion: The patient presented has a T_3 (chest wall involvement) N_0, M_0; stage IIB (per the American Joint Committee on Cancer Staging), non–small-cell lung cancer (NSCLC) of the superior sulcus. Tumors of the superior sulcus represent an uncommon subset of non–small-cell carcinoma. These tumors frequently involve the brachial plexus, subclavian vessels, or spine. Involvement of the brachial plexus causing neuropathic pain radiating down the inner aspect of the arm was first described by Henry Pancoast in 1932. A frequent association is Horner's syndrome consisting of ptosis, miosis, and anhydrosis. It is caused by the invasion of the paravertebral sympathetic chain and the inferior stellate ganglion. Horner's syndrome occurs in 20 to 30% of patients with a superior sulcus tumor.

Staging evaluation of patients with superior sulcus tumors should include complete pulmonary function tests to assess operability, CT scan of the chest through the liver and adrenal glands, a PET scan to exclude distant metastases, a limited MRI of the brachial plexus, and magnetic resonance angiography (MRA) to assess for vessel or brachial plexus involvement.

Preoperative radiation followed by surgical resection became the standard management of NSCLC of the superior sulcus in the 1960s, resulting in a consistent overall survival of approximately 30% at 5 years. Usual contraindications to surgery for superior sulcus tumors include vertebral body invasion, subclavian artery or vein invasion, and clinically evident N_2 disease. More recently, the use of multiple modality therapy with induction chemoradiation and surgical resection has become standard practice. While the goal of preoperative chemotherapy for patients with resectable stage III NSCLC is to eliminate micrometastases, the goal of preoperative chemotherapy plus radiation in the treatment of superior sulcus NSCLC is primarily to shrink down the tumor to improve resectability. In a cooperative group trial reported by Rusch and colleagues, patients with mediastinoscopy-negative T_{3-4} N_{0-1} superior sulcus non–small-cell lung carcinoma received two cycles of cisplatin and etoposide chemotherapy concurrent with 45 Gy of irradiation. Patients with stable or responding disease underwent thoracotomy with *en bloc* resection of the involved lung and chest wall, 3 to 5 weeks later. Induction therapy was completed in 92% of patients with 83 of 111 eligible patients undergoing thoracotomy. Sixty-five percent of thoracotomy specimens showed either pathological complete response or minimal microscopic disease. The 2-year survival was 55% for all eligible patients and 70% for patients who had a complete resection.

The present patient was treated with two cycles of cisplatin and etoposide chemotherapy with concurrent irradiation. He had a partial response to this therapy and successfully underwent a left thoracotomy with a left upper lobectomy. The surgical pathology specimen demonstrated residual microscopic foci of poorly differentiated non–small-cell carcinoma in a background of necrotic pulmonary parenchyma and fibroplasia consistent with marked treatment effect. He has no evidence of recurrent disease 3 months after surgery.

Clinical Pearls

1. Tumors of the superior sulcus may present as Pancoast's syndrome (rib erosion, shoulder pain radiating down the arm, and Horner's syndrome).

2. The use of multiple modality therapy with induction chemoradiation and surgical resection has become standard practice. Downsizing of these tumors with chemotherapy and radiation prior to surgery improves resectability and results in long-term survival in up to 40% of patients.

REFERENCES

1. Jett JR: Superior sulcus tumors and Pancoast's syndrome. Lung Cancer 42:S17-S21, 2003.
2. Pancoast HK: Superior pulmonary sulcus tumor: Tumor characterized by pain, Horner's syndrome, destruction of bone, and atrophy of hand muscles. JAMA 99:1391-1396, 1932.
3. Rusch VW, Giroux DJ, Kraut MJ, et al: Induction chemoradiation and surgical resection for non–small-cell lung carcinomas of the superior sulcus: Initial results of the Southwest Oncology Group trial 9416. J Thorac Cardiovasc Surg 121(3):472-483, 2001.

PATIENT 54

A 58-year-old man with a neck mass

A 58-year-old man presents to his primary physician when he notices a mass in the right side of his neck. The mass does not resolve after a 7-day course of antibiotics, and a fine-needle aspirate reveals squamous cell carcinoma. The patient is referred to an otolaryngologist, whose nasolaryngoscopic examination reveals a tumor on the laryngeal surface of the epiglottis measuring 3 cm in diameter, extending above and below the hyoid bone and to the aryepiglottic folds. A CT scan reveals multiple necrotic lymph nodes in the right neck measuring less than 6 cm, with enlarged lymph nodes measuring less than 2 cm in the left neck. The patient's ENT surgeon has planned primary surgical excision of the supraglottic mass with adjuvant radiation therapy, and the patient presents for a second opinion. The patient reports no hearing deficit or history of renal dysfunction.

Physical Examination: Temperature 36.4°C, pulse 80, respiration 16, blood pressure 140/80 mmHg. General: weight 98.5 kg. HEENT: exophytic lesion measuring approximately 2.5 cm in maximum length on laryngeal surface of epiglottis on mirror examination. Lymph nodes: bulky, ill-defined lymphadenopathy in right anterior cervical triangle; no axillary, supraclavicular, or left cervical lymphadenopathy. Chest: clear bilaterally. Abdomen: soft, nontender, slightly distended, positive bowel sounds. Extremities: no edema.

Radiologic Findings: CT scan of neck: exophytic epiglottic mass (see Figure).

Question: What treatment is the most appropriate for the patient?

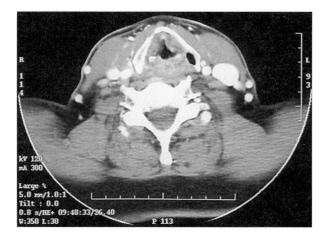

Answer: Concurrent chemoradiation therapy using a platinum-based regimen is the most appropriate treatment.

Discussion: Traditionally, squamous cell carcinoma (SCC) of the head and neck has been managed with primary surgical excision. Cancers determined to be stage I, stage II, and low-bulk stage III by American Joint Committee on Cancer criteria can be cured in 52 to 100% of patients with surgery or radiation therapy alone. Prognosis varies widely depending upon primary site. Although tumors of the glottic larynx present early due to vocal changes, tumors of the adjacent supraglottic larynx are often at an advanced stage on presentation. The tumor in this patient invades the mucosa of more than one adjacent subsite of the supraglottis (T_2), and bilateral lymph nodes measuring less than 6 cm are involved as evidenced by CT and PET scanning (N_2), making this a stage IV disease. Although lymph node involvement decreases cure rates by 50% for any given stage, this patient can still be treated with curative intent because there are no metastatic foci below the clavicle.

Options for treatment include surgical resection, radiation therapy, and chemotherapy alone or in combination. Surgical excision of squamous cell carcinoma in the larynx can, ultimately, require partial or total laryngectomy because clear margins must be established. Such procedures carry a high risk of chronic sequelae, including permanent dysphonia and communication impediment. If a primary surgical approach is employed in patients with bulky stage III and stage IV disease, adjuvant radiation therapy is recommended in most cases to increase the odds of locoregional control and cure.

A Veterans Administration trial compared primary laryngectomy with adjuvant radiation therapy to sequential chemoradiation therapy followed by salvage laryngectomy in patients with laryngeal cancer (the majority with stages III and IV disease). This trial showed no difference in overall survival between the two groups even after 10 years of follow-up, but laryngectomy was avoided in 66% of the patients in the chemoradiation group. This trial established chemoradiation as a larynx-sparing alternative to front-line surgery. A meta-analysis of subsequent studies has shown that platinum-based concomitant chemoradiation confers a statistically significant survival advantage over sequential treatment in patients with nonmetastatic head and neck squamous cell carcinoma. A recent intergroup study supported these findings in patients undergoing concomitant chemoradiation therapy for stages III and IV squamous cancer of the glottic and supraglottic larynx (5-year overall survival was 36%).

In addition to treatment of the primary disease, nodal disease must also be addressed. If a primary surgical approach is pursued, neck dissection can be performed at this time. If chemoradiation is chosen, nodal dissection can be performed before or after therapy, but the latter is generally preferred to ensure that surgical complications do not delay treatment of the primary site. Neck dissection may be avoided in patients with nodal disease less than stage N_2 who have a clinically complete response because radiation alone has been shown to be effective in avoiding recurrence in these patients. Neck dissection may be avoided in selected patients with initially bulky neck disease who have no radiological evidence of nodal disease after chemoradiation therapy. The precise indications of neck dissection in this setting are more controversial, and this represents an active area of investigation.

The present patient went on to receive a 6-week course of external beam radiation. Three cycles of cisplatin and fluorouracil were planned at 21-day intervals during radiation therapy; however, the second cycle was delayed due to neutropenia. The third cycle was not pursued because the delay would have placed its timing after the completion of radiation therapy, when its role as a radiation sensitizer would have been obsolete. Reimaging with CT will be performed approximately 6 weeks after the completion of therapy, with subsequent PET and neck dissection if nodal disease remains. PET scans were delayed until 6 weeks after the completion of therapy, so that the inflammatory treatment effects that may cause false positives will have a chance to resolve.

Clinical Pearls

1. Tumors of the head and neck present at different stages, depending on their primary site, with glottic larynx cancers presenting early and adjacent supraglottic cancers presenting late.

2. Vocal cord paralysis indicates tumor stage no less than T_3.

3. Nodal involvement reduces cure rate by 50% for any given T stage.

4. Platinum-based concomitant chemoradiation therapy offers a larynx-sparing alternative to primary surgical treatment in many cancers of the larynx.

5. Platinum-based chemotherapy increases the efficacy of radiation therapy, but also increases the incidence of severe mucositis and other radiation effects. Many physicians, therefore, place percutaneous gastric feeding tubes before beginning therapy.

REFERENCES

1. Ridge JA, Glisson BS, Horwitz EM, et al: Head and neck tumors. In Pazdur R, Coia LR, Hoskins WJ, Wagman LD (eds): Cancer Management: A Multidisciplinary Approach. New York, CMP Healthcare Media, pp 39-85, 2004.
2. Forastiere AA, Goepfert H, Maor M, et al: Concurrent chemotherapy and radiotherapy for organ preservation in advanced laryngeal cancer. N Engl J Med 349:2091-2098, 2003.
3. Pignon JP, Bourhis J, Domenge C, Designe L: Chemotherapy added to locoregional treatment for head and neck squamous-cell carcinoma: Three meta-analyses of updated individual data. Lancet 355:949-955, 2000.
4. Anonymous: Induction chemotherapy plus radiation compared with surgery plus radiation in patients with advanced laryngeal cancer. The Department of Veterans Affairs Laryngeal Cancer Study Group. N Engl J Med 324(24):1685-1690, 1991.

PATIENT 55

A 69-year-old man with a lung nodule

A 69-year-old man with a history of $T_3N_{2b}M_0$ squamous cell carcinoma of the right base-of-tongue was treated with concurrent platinum-based chemoradiotherapy. He was rendered free of disease. He now returns for routine follow-up 3 years after completing his initial therapy and complains of a new cough. Chest X-ray reveals the interval development of a 2-cm left upper lobe lung nodule. He denies sputum production, hemoptysis, or dyspnea on exertion but does admit to resuming cigarette smoking approximately 2 years previously.

Physical Examination: General: well-appearing, no acute distress. Temperature 36.9°C, blood pressure 120/68 mmHg, pulse 72, weight 78 kg. HEENT: former primary site is clean; no palpable neck, supraclavicular, or axillary adenopathy. Cardiac: regular rate and rhythm, with no murmurs. Chest: clear to auscultation bilaterally. Abdomen: nontender, active bowel sounds, no organomegaly or distention. Extremities: no edema.

Laboratory Findings: Complete blood count, serum chemistry tests, and liver function tests: normal. Chest CT: no additional nodules, abnormal hilar, or mediastinal adenopathy. PET scan: post-treatment changes in neck; lung nodule with standardized uptake value (SUV) of 9.8. Bronchoscopy with transbronchial fine needle aspiration of lung mass: poorly differentiated squamous cell carcinoma cells.

Question: What is the most appropriate next step in management?

Answer: Evaluation for potentially curative surgical resection is the next most appropriate step, because this patient with a history of squamous cell carcinoma of the head and neck has a high probability of having a new primary lung cancer.

Discussion: This patient could have metastatic base-of-tongue cancer, particularly because he had neck node involvement at presentation. However, his long disease-free interval, tobacco history, as well as the solitary lung lesion, are all also consistent with a new early-stage lung carcinoma. This would carry a much better prognosis than distant metastatic disease from head-and-neck cancer. Patients with a history of squamous cell carcinoma of the upper aerodigestive tract are at high risk for second primary cancers, particularly of related body sites also exposed to tobacco and/or alcohol, such as the lung and esophagus. This well-documented "field cancerization effect" leads to an incidence rate of second primary cancers of 3 to 7% per year. The fact that this patient resumed smoking increased his already elevated baseline risk for second malignancy.

There is no consensus on what, if any, routine screening program should be instituted for these patients. Isotretinoin has received considerable attention as a potential chemopreventative agent, but randomized trials have failed to demonstrate a benefit in overall survival.

It is crucial to have this patient evaluated for what could be potentially a curative resection of his solitary lung mass. The most important mistake to avoid is assuming that this patient has an incurable disease.

Clinical Pearls

1. Patients with a history of squamous cell carcinoma of the upper aerodigestive tract are at high risk for second primary cancers, particularly of related body sites also exposed to tobacco and/or alcohol, such as the lung and esophagus.

2. It is crucial to have patients evaluated for what could be potentially a curative resection of a solitary lung mass.

REFERENCE

Yamamoto E, Shibuya H, Yoshimura R, Miura M: Site-specific dependency of second primary cancer in early stage head and neck squamous cell carcinoma. Cancer 94:2007, 2002.

PATIENT 56

A 60-year-old man with locally advanced bladder cancer

A 69-year-old man is referred to a medical oncologist after a urologic evaluation for gross hematuria. A cystoscopy performed 2 weeks prior revealed a firm, nodular mass along the posterior wall of the bladder. The mass was approximately 8 cm and mobile on examination under anesthesia. A transurethral resection of the bladder tumor (TURBT) revealed a high-grade urothelial carcinoma infiltrating into the muscularis propria. The exam under anesthesia revealed the bladder to be mobile. No lymphadenopathy or distant metastases were detected on a CT scan of the abdomen and pelvis. A chest X-ray revealed no abnormal findings.

Past medical history is significant for thalassemia trait. Family history is negative for malignancy. Social history is notable for a 20-pack-year history of cigarette smoking. The patient notes urinary frequency, urgency, and intermittent hematuria.

Physical Examination: Temperature 36.1°C, pulse 60, blood pressure 120/70 mmHg. General: well-appearing, no acute distress. HEENT: no scleral icterus, mucous membranes moist. Neck: no adenopathy. Cardiovascular: regular rate and rhythm, without murmurs. Chest: clear to auscultation bilaterally. Abdomen: soft, nontender, no organomegaly or masses. Extremities: no axillary adenopathy, edema, or calf tenderness.

Laboratory Findings: Hemoglobin 10.1 g/dL, WBC 7900/µL, platelets 343,000/µL, creatinine 1.1 mg/dL.

Questions: Is neoadjuvant chemotherapy indicated? If so, which chemotherapy regimen is recommended? What is the appropriate surgical intervention?

Answers: The patient should be offered neoadjuvant chemotherapy. Neoadjuvant cisplatin-based combination chemotherapy has been shown to improve survival in patients with clinical stage T_2-T_{4a} transitional cell carcinoma of the bladder compared to surgery alone. Following 3 months of chemotherapy, the patient should undergo a radical cystoprostatectomy with an "adequate" lymph node dissection.

Discussion: The patient has clinical stage $T_2N_0M_0$ transitional cell carcinoma (TCC) of the bladder. Although his disease is currently surgically resectable, approximately 50% of patients with invasive TCC will develop metastases and die. Given the chemosensitivity of TCC, attempts to improve survival have focused on administering chemotherapy in the perioperative setting.

Over the past decade, multiple trials have explored neoadjuvant chemotherapy in TCC. Several of these studies failed to show a benefit for chemotherapy; however, many suffered from inadequate sample size, suboptimal chemotherapeutic regimens, premature closure, or inadequate follow-up time. Recently, well-designed prospective trials and a meta-analysis have shifted the treatment paradigm in muscle-invasive disease toward the use of neoadjuvant chemotherapy.

Intergroup trial 0080 randomized 317 patients with clinical stage T_2-T_{4a} TCC of the bladder to radical cystectomy alone versus three cycles of methotrexate, vinblastine, doxorubicin, and cisplatin (MVAC) followed by radical cystectomy. The use of neoadjuvant chemotherapy was associated with a higher rate of complete pathological response (38% vs 15%, $p < 0.001$) and 5-year survival (57% vs 43%, $p = 0.06$). In a recently published meta-analysis of 2688 patients treated in ten randomized trials evaluating neoadjuvant chemotherapy for invasive TCC (not including data from Intergroup 0080), neoadjuvant platinum-based combination chemotherapy was associated with a significant benefit in overall survival (HR = 0.98 [95% CI, 0.78-0.98, $p = 0.016$]), a 13% decrease in the risk of death, and a 5% absolute survival benefit at 5 years (overall survival increased from 45-50%).

Following chemotherapy, the patient should undergo a radical cystoprostatectomy and lymph node dissection. This holds true even for patients achieving a complete clinical response (on repeat cystoscopy), because there is a marked discordance between clinical and pathological responses (upon evaluation of cystectomy specimen). The importance of an "adequate" pelvic lymph node dissection cannot be underscored. Three retrospective studies have correlated improved survival with an increased number of lymph nodes removed at surgery in both patients with pN_0 and pN_1 disease. Adequate lymphadenectomy was defined as at least 11 to 16 nodes in these studies. The optimal number of lymph nodes removed has not yet been established.

The data detailed earlier support the use of neoadjuvant cisplatin-based combination chemotherapy in patients with invasive urothelial TCC. Although MVAC is a treatment standard, the use of gemcitabine plus cisplatin (GC) has been adopted by some oncologists because GC showed comparable response and survival to MVAC in a randomized trial of patients with metastatic disease. The former regimen was also associated with substantially less toxicity. Neoadjuvant chemotherapy should be administered for 3 months. There are no current data to support the use of carboplatin-based regimens in the perioperative setting.

As a consequence of small sample size, inclusion of heterogenous populations of patients with muscle-invasive disease, and potentially inadequate chemotherapy, the data supporting the use of adjuvant chemotherapy are less compelling than those supporting neoadjuvant chemotherapy. Two small trials of cisplatin-based therapy have shown a survival benefit leading many oncologists to recommend adjuvant chemotherapy, if there is pathological evidence of extra vesicular or node-positive disease following cystectomy. However, to definitively address this issue, two large cooperative group trials are underway.

In the present patient, three cycles of GC were administered, followed by a radical cystoprostatectomy. The patient remains without evidence of recurrent disease at 2 years follow-up.

Clinical Pearls

1. Recurrent/metastatic disease will develop in large proportion of patients who undergo radical cystectomy for invasive transitional cell carcinoma.

2. Perioperative cisplatin-based combination chemotherapy improves survival in patients with invasive transitional cell carcinoma (TCC). Given the limitations of several completed trials, the data are more compelling for neoadjuvant chemotherapy than adjuvant chemotherapy.

3. There is currently no role for carboplatin-based combination chemotherapy in the perioperative setting. Therefore, patients with contraindications to cisplatin (e.g., inadequate renal function) should not receive perioperative chemotherapy outside of a clinical trial.

4. An increased number of lymph nodes removed at the time of surgery has been correlated with improved survival.

REFERENCES

1. Grossman HB, Natale RB, Tangen CM, et al: Neoadjuvant chemotherapy plus cystectomy compared with cystectomy alone for locally advanced bladder cancer. N Engl J Med 349:859-866, 2003.
2. Herr HW: Extent of surgery and pathology evaluation has an impact on bladder cancer outcomes after radical cystectomy. Urology 61:105-108, 2003.
3. Konety BR, Joslyn SA, O'Donnell MA: Extent of pelvic lymphadenectomy and its impact on outcome in patients diagnosed with bladder cancer: Analysis of data from the Surveillance, Epidemiology and End Results Program data base. J Urol 169:946-950, 2003.
4. Neoadjuvant chemotherapy in invasive bladder cancer: A systematic review and meta-analysis. Lancet 361:1927-1934, 2003.
5. von der Maase H, Hansen SW, Roberts JT, et al: Gemcitabine and cisplatin versus methotrexate, vinblastine, doxorubicin, and cisplatin in advanced or metastatic bladder cancer: Results of a large, randomized, multinational, multicenter, phase III study. J Clin Oncol 18:3068-3077, 2000.
6. Studer UE, Bacchi M, Biedermann C, et al: Adjuvant cisplatin chemotherapy following cystectomy for bladder cancer: Results of a prospective randomized trial. J Urol l152:81-84, 1994.
7. Skinner DG, Daniels JR, Russell CA, et al: The role of adjuvant chemotherapy following cystectomy for invasive bladder cancer: A prospective comparative trial. J Urol 145:459-464; discussion 464-467, 1991.

PATIENT 57

A 52-year-old woman with hematuria

A previously healthy 52-year-old woman presents with gross hematuria. She denies any other symptoms. She specifically denies fevers, weight loss, and pain in her abdomen, flank, or pelvis.

Physical Examination: General: well-appearing, no acute distress. Karnofsky performance status: 90%. Vital signs: blood pressure 124/80 mmHg, pulse 64, respirations 12, temperature 36.9°C. HEENT: no scleral icterus, mucous membranes moist; neck supple, no adenopathy. Cardiac: regular rate and rhythm, without murmurs. Chest: clear to auscultation bilaterally, no wheezing or rales. Breasts: no palpable masses, no discharge. Abdomen: soft, nontender, no organomegaly or masses. Lymph nodes: no peripheral adenopathy. Extremities: no edema.

Laboratory Findings: Electrolytes: normal. BUN 15 mg/dL, creatinine 0.7 mg/dL, hemoglobin 14.5 g/dL, platelets 240 K/mcL, LDH 128 U/L, alkaline phosphatase 73 U/L. Urine cytology: positive for malignant cells. Cystoscopy: 5-cm sessile lesion involving right urethral orifice. Transurethral resection of bladder tumor: high-grade urothelial carcinoma invading muscularis propria; 4+ overexpression of p53. Staging CT scan of chest, abdomen (see Figure), and pelvis: significant retroperitoneal adenopathy measuring 2.5 cm in greatest dimension. Bone scan: no evidence of osseous metastases.

Questions: At what stage is the patient's disease? What is the recommended management?

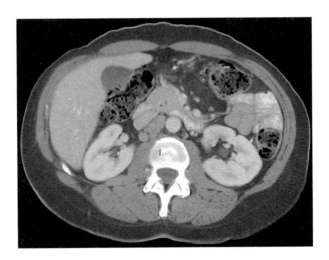

Answers: This patient has clinical stage $T_2N_2M_0$ high-grade urothelial carcinoma of the bladder. Given her extensive lymphadenopathy on CT scan, she has stage IV disease and is therefore not a candidate for up-front radical cystectomy. Chemotherapy is the approach of choice in unresectable metastatic bladder cancer.

Discussion: Of the 25% of bladder cancers that are muscle-invasive at the time of diagnosis, almost 50% will harbor metastatic or micrometastatic disease. Nearly 50% of patients who undergo a radical cystectomy as primary therapy for muscle-invasive disease will relapse with metastases within 2 years. Common sites of metastasis include regional and distant lymph nodes, bone, lung, liver, and skin.

Bladder cancer is chemosensitive. In the metastatic setting, overall response rates range from 12 to 73%, with complete responses of 0 to 36%. Cisplatin is the most active agent; other active agents include ifosfamide, cyclophosphamide, carboplatin, doxorubicin, paclitaxel, docetaxel, methotrexate, gemcitabine, and vinblastine.

Median survival for metastatic disease treated with single-agent chemotherapy is less than 6 months. Higher response rates and improvement in median survival are reported with combination chemotherapy regimens that include cisplatin. Methotrexate, vinblastine, doxorubicin, cisplatin (MVAC) is the standard of care for unresectable or metastatic bladder cancer, with median survival of approximately 1 year and 3 to 7% of patients achieving long-term survival.

MVAC has been found superior in phase III trials to single-agent cisplatin or to the combination of cisplatin, cyclophosphamide plus doxorubicin. High-dose accelerated MVAC (2-week cycle) with G-CSF support increases the proportion of complete responses but does not impact overall survival. There is significant toxicity associated with MVAC, and toxic death rates are 3 to 9%. G-CSF support improves the associated hematological toxicities.

Pretreatment risk factors associated with worse outcomes in metastatic bladder cancer treated with chemotherapy include poor performance status (Karnofsky Performance Status [KPS] $\leq$ 80) and the presence of visceral metastases (lung, liver, bone). Median survival and probability of 5-year survival vary based on these factors:

Risk Factors	Median Survival	5-yr Survival
0	33 months	33%
1	13 months	11%
2	9 months	0%

Other predictors of worse chemotherapy response rate and survival include weight loss,

nontransitional cell carcinoma histology, expression of the multidrug resistance gene, p53 overexpression, increased serum alkaline phosphatase, and increased LDH levels.

Promising new regimens have demonstrated comparable efficacy to MVAC with fewer toxicities. A phase III study compared MVAC to GC. Response rates and survival were similar, but GC was better tolerated. Ifosfamide, paclitaxel, plus cisplatin (ITP) has demonstrated a 68% overall response rate and median survival of 20 months and is well-tolerated. A phase III trial of this regimen with the addition of sequential doxorubicin and gemcitabine (AG-ITP) reported a 43% complete remission rate.

Carboplatin has been substituted for cisplatin in several phase II trials, and a head-to-head comparison was reported by Dogliotti and colleagues at the 2003 American Society of Clinical Oncology meeting. This study compared cisplatin–gemcitabine to carboplatin–gemcitabine in advanced or metastatic bladder cancer, with no statistically significant difference in toxicity, similar overall response rate, but lower complete response rate with carboplatin. Until additional evidence is available, carboplatin-based regimens should be restricted to patients in whom cure is not likely or when cisplatin therapy is not feasible.

The role of surgery in metastatic bladder cancer is not well established. Surgery is considered for patients whose disease is restricted to the pelvis or regional lymph nodes and in those who demonstrate a major response to chemotherapy. In a series at Memorial Sloan-Kettering Cancer Center, 207 patients with unresectable disease received chemotherapy; 80 then underwent surgical resection. Pathological complete remission was found in 30%, with 61% demonstrating residual viable cancer, which was then completely resected, yielding a 91% complete remission rate. Surgery for limited distant metastases in selected patients was reported from MD Anderson: 30 of 31 patients (97%) were rendered disease-free following metastasectomy of the lung (77%), distant lymph nodes (13%), brain (7%), or subcutaneous tissues (3%), with 33% 5-year survival.

The present patient had 0 of 2 poor prognostic risk factors (KPS 90%, no visceral metastases). Her best chance for long-term survival was therapy with a cisplatin-based regimen, such as MVAC, GC, or an experimental protocol. The addition of surgery after a major response to chemotherapy could contribute to her chance of cure. She decided to enroll in a protocol using sequential AG-ITP and experienced a clinical complete response, evidenced by resolution of lymphadenopathy on abdominal CT scan (see Figure, below). She then underwent an anterior exenteration, including radical cystectomy, total abdominal hysterectomy, bilateral salpingo-oophorectomy, extended bilateral pelvic lymph node dissection, and Indiana pouch construction for urinary diversion. Surgical pathology revealed no residual disease. She is now nearly 4 years post-treatment with no evidence of disease.

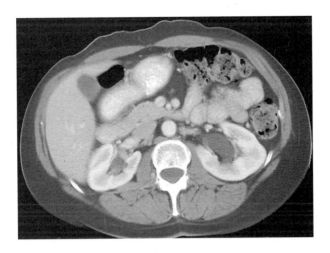

Clinical Pearls

1. Standard chemotherapy regimens in unresectable or metastatic bladder cancer include cisplatin, such as MVAC or GC. If cisplatin cannot be given or cure is not feasible, carboplatin may be substituted.

2. Pretreatment predictors of worse outcome include poor performance status and visceral metastases.

3. Surgery may play a role for resection of regional disease in complete remission following chemotherapy, or for metastasectomy of limited distant metastases.

REFERENCES

1. Siefker-Radtke AO, Walsh GL, Pisters LL, et al: Is there a role for surgery in the management of metastatic urothelial cancer? The M. D. Anderson experience. J Urol 171(1):145-148, 2004.
2. Hussain SA, James ND: The systemic treatment of advanced and metastatic bladder cancer. Lancet Oncol 4(8):489-497, 2003.
3. Juffs HG, Moore MJ, Tannock IF: The role of systemic chemotherapy in the management of muscle-invasive bladder cancer. Lancet Oncol 3(12):738-747, 2002.
4. Herr HW, Donat SM, Bajorin DF: Post-chemotherapy surgery in patients with unresectable or regionally metastatic bladder cancer. J Urol 165(3):811-814, 2001.
5. Sternberg CN, de Mulder PH, Schornagel JH, et al: Randomized phase III trial of high-dose-intensity methotrexate, vinblastine, doxorubicin, and cisplatin (MVAC) chemotherapy and recombinant human granulocyte colony-stimulating factor versus classic MVAC in advanced urothelial tract tumors: European Organization for Research and Treatment of Cancer Protocol no. 30924. J Clin Oncol 19(10):2638-2646, 2001.
6. Bajorin DF, McCaffrey JA, Dodd PM, et al: Ifosfamide, paclitaxel, and cisplatin for patients with advanced transitional cell carcinoma of the urothelial tract: Final report of a phase II trial evaluating two dosing schedules. Cancer 88(7):1671-1678, 2000.
7. von der Maase H, Hansen SW, Roberts JT, et al: Gemcitabine and cisplatin versus methotrexate, vinblastine, doxorubicin, and cisplatin in advanced or metastatic bladder cancer: Results of a large, randomized, multinational, multicenter, phase III study. J Clin Oncol 18(17):3068-3077, 2000.
8. Bajorin DF, Dodd PM, Mazumdar M, et al: Long-term survival in metastatic transitional-cell carcinoma and prognostic factors predicting outcome of therapy. J Clin Oncol 17(10):3173-3181, 1999.
9. Saxman SB, Propert KJ, Einhorn LH, et al: Long-term follow-up of a phase III intergroup study of cisplatin alone or in combination with methotrexate, vinblastine, and doxorubicin in patients with metastatic urothelial carcinoma: A cooperative group study. J Clin Oncol 15(7):2564-2569, 1997.

10. Bales GT, Kim H, Steinberg GD: Surgical therapy for locally advanced bladder cancer. Semin Oncol 23(5):605-613, 1996.
11. Sternberg CN, Yagoda A, Scher HI, et al: Methotrexate, vinblastine, doxorubicin, and cisplatin for advanced transitional cell carcinoma of the urothelium. Efficacy and patterns of response and relapse. Cancer 64(12):2448-2458, 1989.
12. Whitmore WF Jr: Management of invasive bladder neoplasms. Semin Urol 1(1):34-41, 1983.

PATIENT 58

A 29-year-old man with pulmonary nodules

A 29-year-old man was initially diagnosed with a nonseminomatous germ cell tumor (NSGCT) involving his right testicle. A staging CT scan demonstrated an inter-aortocaval lymph node measuring 2.2 cm in size, and his tumor markers included β-hCG less than 2 U/mL (normal < 5), alpha-fetoprotein (AFP) 6.0 ng/mL (normal < 6.1), and LDH 135 U/L (normal 100–250). He was therefore considered to be good risk, clinical stage IIB. He was treated with four cycles of etoposide–cisplatin (EP) followed by retroperitoneal lymph node dissection. Pathology demonstrated viable residual embryonal carcinoma in 3 of 14 lymph nodes, and he therefore received two additional cycles of EP. He was followed with a monthly physical exam, chest X-ray, and tumor marker levels. He now returns for a 4-month follow-up appointment.

Physical Examination: General: well-appearing, no acute distress. Karnofsky performance status: 90%. Blood pressure 100/70 mmHg, pulse 60, respirations 16, temperature 36.6°C. HEENT: no scleral icterus, mucous membranes moist; neck supple, no adenopathy. Cardiac: regular rate and rhythm, without murmurs. Chest: clear to auscultation bilaterally, no wheezing or rales. Breasts: no gynecomastia or tenderness to palpation. Abdomen: soft, nontender, no organomegaly or masses. Genitourinary: remaining testis nontender, without masses. Lymph nodes: no peripheral adenopathy. Extremities: no edema.

Laboratory Findings: Complete blood count and serum chemistries: normal. LDH 123 U/L, β-hCG < 2 U/mL, AFP 2 ng/mL. Chest X-ray and CT scan: multiple pulmonary nodules suspicious for metastatic disease (see Figures). CT-guided biopsy of lung nodule: recurrent metastatic embryonal carcinoma.

Question: Is this patient potentially curable?

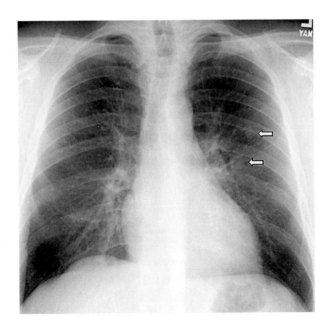

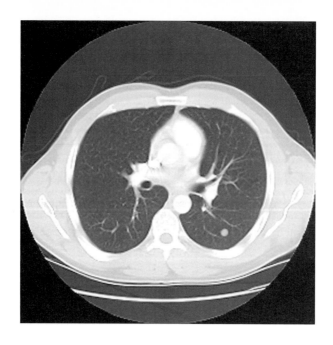

Answer: Even in a setting of recurrent metastatic NSGCT, there is a potential for cure.

Discussion: Between 5 and 20% of patients with metastatic germ cell tumors of the testis will relapse after primary chemotherapy, depending on whether or not viable residual disease is found at retroperitoneal lymph node dissection. Most relapses occur within 2 years of completing treatment. "Late relapse" (not discussed here) by definition occurs at greater than 2 years after completing primary therapy.

Most cases of residual or recurrent disease are detected by tumor markers or imaging studies, and elevations of serum tumor markers are the most sensitive means of detecting early relapse. A rising AFP and/or β-hCG without clinical findings or radiographic evidence implies residual or relapsed disease and is sufficient to justify treatment, as long as other causes of elevated tumor markers have been ruled out. An enlarging mass in the setting of normal serum markers suggests a growing teratoma, which should be managed surgically. PET imaging has demonstrated a high positive predictive value in determining viable residual seminoma in post-chemotherapy residual tumors greater than 3 cm in size. Unfortunately, PET cannot detect teratoma or reliably detect disease in small nodes in patients with NSGCT. Therefore, the usefulness of PET is very limited.

Several factors should be considered when selecting appropriate second-line therapy for relapsed disease: site of primary disease, initial therapy response and duration, location of recurrence, and histology. Factors that are associated

with a favorable outcome to standard dose salvage chemotherapy include a testis primary site and complete response to initial treatment. Standard therapy for patients who relapse after a complete remission includes an ifosfamide and cisplatin-containing regimen. A combination of vinblastine, ifosfamide, and cisplatin (VeIP) has been used as salvage therapy when etoposide was included in the primary regimen. Using ifosfamide and cisplatin-containing regimens, approximately 35% of patients will obtain a complete remission and 25% can be cured. More recently, a 77% complete remission rate and 85% 2-year survival has been reported using paclitaxel, ifosfamide, and cisplatin (TIP) in relapsed patients with favorable characteristics. There are no reliable phase III data comparing VeIP to TIP.

Patients with less favorable prognostic factors, such as a mediastinal primary site and/or incomplete response to initial therapy, should be considered for clinical trials, including dose-intensive therapies. Approximately 5 to 20% of cisplatin-resistant patients can be cured with two cycles of high-dose carboplatin given with etoposide and cyclophosphamide followed by stem cell rescue. Other chemotherapy agents that have demonstrated activity in cisplatin-refractory disease include etoposide, ifosfamide, paclitaxel, gemcitabine, and, more recently, oxaliplatin.

The present patient was found to have a primary good risk NSGCT originating in the testis, for which he initially received etoposide and cisplatin (EP). He experienced a complete remission that lasted 4 months, followed by disease recurrence in the lungs. Possible treatments, given his favorable predictors, now include either VeIP (because he had etoposide previously) or TIP.

Clinical Pearls

1. Recurrent nonseminomatous germ cell tumor is potentially curable.
2. Favorable response to salvage chemotherapy is associated with a testis primary site and a prior complete response to primary chemotherapy.

REFERENCES

1. De Santis M, Becherer A, Bokemeyer C: 2-18 fluoro-deoxy-D-glucose positron emission tomography is a reliable predictor for viable tumor in postchemotherapy seminoma: An update of the prospective multicentric SEMPET trial. J Clin Oncol 22(6):1034-1039, 2004.
2. Kollmannsberger C, Beyer J, Liersch R, et al: Combination chemotherapy with gemcitabine plus oxaliplatin in patients with intensively pretreated or refractory germ cell cancer: A study of the German Testicular Cancer Study Group. J Clin Oncol 22(1):108-114, 2004.
3. Motzer RJ, Sheinfeld J, Mazumdar M: Paclitaxel, ifosfamide, and cisplatin second-line therapy for patients with relapsed testicular germ cell cancer. J Clin Oncol 18(12):2413-2418, 2000.
4. Bokemeyer C, Gerl A, Schoffski P: Gemcitabine in patients with relapsed or cisplatin-refractory testicular cancer. J Clin Oncol 17(2):512-516, 1999.
5. Loehrer PJ Sr, Gonin R, Nichols CR, et al: Vinblastine plus ifosfamide plus cisplatin as initial salvage therapy in recurrent germ cell tumor. J Clin Oncol 16(7):2500-2504, 1998.
6. McCaffrey JA, Mazumdar M, Bajorin DF, et al: Ifosfamide- and cisplatin-containing chemotherapy as first-line salvage therapy in germ cell tumors: Response and survival. J Clin Oncol 15(7):2559-2563, 1997.
7. Motzer RJ, Bajorin DF, Schwartz LH, et al: Phase II trial of paclitaxel shows antitumor activity in patients with previously treated germ cell tumors. J Clin Oncol 12(11):2277-2283, 1994.
8. Motzer RJ, Bosl GJ: High-dose chemotherapy for resistant germ cell tumors: Recent advances and future directions. J Natl Cancer Inst 84(22):1703-1709, 1992.
9. Harstrick A, Schmoll HJ, Wilke H: Cisplatin, etoposide, and ifosfamide salvage therapy for refractory or relapsing germ cell carcinoma. J Clin Oncol 9(9):1549-1555, 1991.
10. Toner GC, Geller NL, Tan C, et al: Serum tumor marker half-life during chemotherapy allows early prediction of complete response and survival in nonseminomatous germ cell tumors. Cancer Res 50(18):5904-5910, 1990.

PATIENT 59

A 26-year-old man with a left testicular mass

A 26-year-old man presents with a 3-month history of a painless left testicular mass. An ultrasound reveals a 3 cm × 2.2 cm mass in the left testicle. Three days later, the patient is taken to the operating room for a left inguinal orchiectomy. Surgical pathology reveals a teratoma limited to the testis (pT$_1$). The patient is now 1 week post-surgery. He denies back pain, cough, dyspnea, or nipple tenderness.

Physical Examination: General: well-appearing. Blood pressure 110/70 mmHg, temperature 37°C. HEENT: no scleral icterus, mucous membranes moist, no adenopathy. Cardiovascular: regular rate and rhythm, without murmurs. Chest: clear to auscultation bilaterally, no gynecomastia. Abdomen: soft, nontender, no organomegaly or masses. Genitourinary: left inguinal incision site healing well, right testicle with no palpable masses. Extremities: no axillary adenopathy, edema, or calf tenderness.

Laboratory Findings: Prior to orchiectomy: LDH 159 U/L (normal 100–250), β-HCG < 2 U/mL (normal < 2.2), alpha-fetoprotein (AFP) 4.6 ng/mL (normal < 15). CT scan of chest, abdomen, and pelvis: bilateral 1-cm pulmonary nodules and multiple necrotic left paraaortic lymph nodes measuring up to 3 cm (see Figures).

Questions: What is the diagnosis? How should patient be risk stratified? What is the appropriate treatment plan?

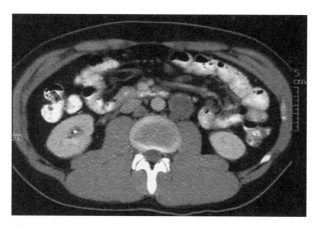

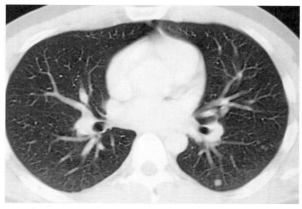

Answers: Despite the presence of only teratoma in the orchiectomy specimen, the patient has a fully malignant nonseminomatous germ cell tumor (NSGCT). There is radiographic evidence of metastases to the retroperitoneal lymph nodes and lungs. Based on the International Germ Cell Cancer Collaborative Group (IGCCCG) Consensus Classification, the patient has good risk disease. He should receive four cycles of etoposide plus cisplatin (EP) or three cycles of bleomycin, etoposide, and cisplatin (BEP). Following chemotherapy, all residual abnormalities should be resected.

Discussion: Germ cell tumors develop from primitive germ cells and are classified as either seminoma or nonseminoma. Embryonal carcinoma, the most undifferentiated cell type of the nonseminomatous germ cell tumors, has the capacity to differentiate into the other nonseminomatous cells types: teratoma, choriocarcinoma, and yolk-sac carcinoma. Therefore, the presence of pure teratoma in the pathology specimen of a post-pubertal male implies the presence of, and mandates the treatment for, a fully malignant NSGCT.

Correct classification of germ cell tumors is necessary because the clinical management of seminoma and nonseminoma differs. Sometimes, both seminomatous and nonseminomatous elements are present in the pathology specimen, in which case management should follow that for nonseminotamous tumors. Serum β-HCG may be elevated in either seminoma or nonseminoma, but AFP is elevated in nonseminoma only. Therefore, if the AFP is elevated, even if pathology reveals pure seminoma, the patient should be treated for an NSGCT.

Primary chemotherapy after orchiectomy is warranted for all patients with NSGCT with persistently elevated tumor markers even in the absence of radiographic abnormalities (stage I-S disease), retroperitoneal lymph node metastases greater than 5 cm (stage IIC disease), multiple retroperitoneal lymph nodes, distant metastases (stage III disease), or tumor-related back pain. Primary chemotherapy is also indicated for all patients with extragonadal primary tumors. Patients with solitary nodal disease of 2 to 5 cm and negative markers may sometimes receive chemotherapy and sometimes surgery, depending on specific circumstances.

This patient has multiple enlarged retroperitoneal lymph nodes in the primary nodal landing zone for left-sided testis tumors (paraaortic region; left testicular vein drains into the left renal vein). In addition, there are findings consistent with pulmonary metastases. This patient should receive primary chemotherapy.

All patients requiring primary chemotherapy should be risk stratified according to the IGCCCG classification. This classification scheme, based on a multivariate analysis of prognostic factors in more than 5000 patients, includes the primary tumor site (testicular or retroperitoneal vs mediastinal), degree of serum tumor marker elevation, and the presence of nonpulmonary visceral metastases. In the analysis, three prognostic groupings were developed based on these factors: good risk (91% 5-year survival), intermediate risk (79% 5-year survival), and poor risk (48% 5-year survival). These strata are incorporated into the American Joint Committee on Cancer/Union Internationale Contre le Cancer staging classification for germ cell tumors (GCT). This patient with a testicular primary tumor, normal serum markers, and no evidence of non-pulmonary visceral metastases, has good risk disease.

The available data support the initial use of either four cycles of etoposide plus cisplatin (EP) or three cycles of bleomycin, etoposide, and cisplatin (BEP) for patients with good risk disease. Recently, the preliminary results of a French randomized trial comparing these two regimens showed no significant difference in overall survival. Omission of bleomycin is attractive given the potential for Raynaud's phenomenon and pulmonary toxicity. Patients with intermediate or poor risk should be treated with four cycles of BEP or enrolled in a clinical trial.

Following chemotherapy for NSGCT, all sites of residual abnormalities should be resected (assuming markers have normalized). In the retroperitoneum, 45 to 50% of residual masses will be necrotic debris/fibrosis, 35 to 40% will be teratoma, and 10 to 20% will be viable GCT. Resection of teratoma is critical given the risk for residual viable GCT, late relapse, and/or malignant transformation. If viable GCT is found, patients should receive two additional cycles of EP.

Clinical Pearls

1. Patients with pure teratoma, pure seminoma with elevated serum AFP, or mixed seminoma/nonseminoma all have, and should be treated for, nonseminomatous germ cell tumor (NSGCT).

2. Patients with NSGCT requiring primary chemotherapy should be risk stratified, because treatment recommendations differ according to risk group.

3. Post-chemotherapy surgery of residual abnormalities is an integral component of a curative treatment program for NSGCT, given the risk of a persistent teratoma or viable tumor.

REFERENCES

1. Bosl GJ, Bajorin DF, Sheinfeld J, et al: Cancer of the testis. In Devita VT, Hellman S, Rosenberg SA (eds): Cancer: Principles and Practices of Oncology, 7th ed. Philadelphia, Lippincott, Williams & Wilkins, 2004.

2. Culine S, Kerbrat P, Bouzy J, et al: The optimal chemotherapy regimen for good-risk metastatic non seminomatous germ cell tumors (MNSGCT) is 3 cycles of bleomycin, etoposide and cisplatin: Mature results of a randomized trial. Proc Am Soc Clin Oncol Abstract 1536, 2003.

3. Fizazi K, Tjulandin S, Salvioni R, et al: Viable malignant cells after primary chemotherapy for disseminated nonseminomatous germ cell tumors: Prognostic factors and role of postsurgery chemotherapy—Results from an international study group. J Clin Oncol 19:2647-2657, 2001.

4. International Germ Cell Consensus Classification: A prognostic factor-based staging system for metastatic germ cell cancers. International Germ Cell Cancer Collaborative Group. J Clin Oncol 15:594-603, 1997.

5. Vogelzang NJ, Bosl GJ, Johnson K, et al: Raynaud's phenomenon: A common toxicity after combination chemotherapy for testicular cancer. Ann Intern Med 95:288-292, 1981.

PATIENT 60

A 53-year-old man with right upper quadrant pain

A 53-year-old man with a past medical history significant for seminomatous testicular cancer, orchiectomy and chemotherapy, and early-stage esophageal cancer post Ivor-Lewis esophagectomy presents to the emergency department complaining of 4 days of increasing right upper quadrant pain and fever. A CT scan shows inflammation of the large and small bowel as well as a thickened appendix. He is taken to the operating room for emergent appendectomy.

Physical Examination: Temperature 37°C, pulse 107, blood pressure 120/73 mmHg. HEENT: sclerae anicteric, no adenopathy. Cardiac: regular rate and rhythm, without murmurs. Chest: clear. Abdomen: soft, bowel sounds present, no masses felt, colostomy in place, multiple old and new abdominal scars. Genital exam: implant in left testicle. Extremities: significant left lower extremity edema.

Laboratory Findings: WBC 5700/μL, hemoglobin 15.4 g/dL, platelets 202/μL. Electrolytes: normal. Pathology appendectomy specimen: acute appendicitis and abscess formation, glandular cells with signet ring features, and a minor component of goblet cells. Focal positivity for chromogranin and synaptophysin.

Questions: What is the most likely diagnosis? What is the treatment for this condition?

Answers: Adenocarcinoma of the appendix is the most likely diagnosis. The treatment is right hemicolectomy.

Discussion: Adenocarcinoma of the appendix is a spectrum of diseases. Epithelial tumors of the appendix have been classified into four distinct types: carcinoids, mucinous adenocarcinoma, colonic-type adenocarcinoma, and adeno carcinoids. Carcinoid tumors account for 85% of the epithelial appendiceal tumors. A mucinous adenocarcinoma can be distinguished from the much rarer colonic-type adenocarcinoma of the appendix in that at least 50% of the lesion is composed of mucin. The tumor tends to be more diffuse and forms mucoceles. Most adenocarcinomas of the appendix evolve probably through an adenoma-carcinoma sequence, similar to other colonic neoplasms.

Primary appendiceal adenocarcinoma accounts for less then 0.5% of all gastrointestinal tumors and 5% of primary appendiceal neoplasms. The most common clinical presentation of primary appendiceal adenocarcinoma is a palpable mass or acute appendicitis. Rarely is the diagnosis of a primary appendiceal adenocarcinoma made preoperatively, because neither abdominal ultrasound nor CT can differentiate between this and other conditions. Even intraoperatively the diagnosis is only considered in a third of cases. Adenocarcinomas of the appendix are frequently misdiagnosed as ovarian cancer, metastatic adenocarcinoma of unknown primary, ruptured appendix, hernia, or ileocecal colon cancer. The mean age for appendiceal neoplasm is 56 years, and there is a slight male predominance. Histologically, CK-20 positivity is consistent with gastrointestinal origin, while CK-7 is generally attributed to gynecological tumors. However, appendiceal carcinomas can be CK-7 positive in 50% of patients.

Treatment and prognosis depend on the most aggressive cell type found in the pathology specimen. The anatomical peculiarities of the appendix lead to several considerations in regard to appendiceal neoplasm. The narrow appendiceal diameter predisposes to occlusion of the lumen by the tumor early in its course. Another anatomical consideration is that the appendix often has deficiencies of both longitudinal and circular muscle fibers, which predispose to perforation and also lead to early dissemination. The most common metastatic location is the peritoneal cavity, followed by lymph nodes, liver, ovaries, abdominal wall, and lungs. Second primary synchronous and metachronous neoplasms, especially in the GI tract, are found in up to 35% of patients with appendix adenocarcinoma. A search for either a synchronous or a metachronous neoplasm should be performed during follow-up.

Patients who had a right hemicolectomy have a better prognosis for survival than those with appendectomy only. The prognosis of adenocarcinoma of the appendix is determined by Duke's stage, and is similar, stage by stage, to that of colorectal carcinoma. Adenocarcinomas of the appendix behave differently from other colorectal cancers. They have a predilection for peritoneal surfaces and rarely metastasize to other visceral organs. Their treatment also differs from the treatment of the other colorectal cancers. Right hemicolectomy is the standard of care. For peritoneal disease, debulking to deposits of less than 5 mm is indicated, if feasible. Intraperitoneal chemotherapy is administered when disease can be optimally debulked. The value of intraperitoneal chemotherapy in the setting of large-volume intraperitoneal disease is less certain. Largely because this is a rare tumor with protean manifestations and several different histological subtypes, data from prospective randomized controlled trials are lacking. For example, there are no large randomized clinical trials comparing systemic versus intraperitoneal for advanced appendiceal cancers. Recent studies evaluating the role of aggressive debulking surgery are suggesting a benefit.

The present patient received six cycles of FOLFOX (5-FU, leucovorin, and oxaliplatin). Repeat imaging studies revealed no evidence of disease. He was then taken to the operating room for a completion right hemicolectomy. At surgery, the patient was found to have peritoneal carcinomatosis that could not be optimally debulked. He is presently receiving 5-FU, leucovorin, and irinotecan (FOLFIRI) chemotherapy for metastatic disease.

Clinical Pearls

1. The most common presentation of appendiceal adenocarcinoma is a ruptured appendix.

2. Adenocarcinomas of the appendix are associated with long-standing inflammatory bowel disease and other autoimmune diseases.

3. Adenocarcinoma of the appendix behaves similarly to ovarian cancer with a predilection for peritoneal surfaces, and visceral metastases are rare.

4. Standard therapy for appendiceal adenocarcinoma is right hemicolectomy.

REFERENCES

1. Lo NS, Sarr MG: Mucinous cystadenoma of the appendix. The controversy persists: A review. Hepatogastroenterology 50:432-457, 2003.
2. Ozakyol AH, Saricam T, Kabukcuoglu S, et al: Primary appendiceal adenocarcinoma. Am J Clin Oncol 22:458-459, 1999.
3. Cortina R, McCormick J, Kolm P, Perry RR: Management and prognosis of adenocarcinoma of the appendix. Dis Colon Rectum 38:848-852, 1995.
4. Deans GT, Spence RA: Neoplastic lesions of the appendix. Br J Surg 82:299-306, 1995.
5. Sugarbaker PH: Patient selection and treatment of peritoneal carcinomatosis from colorectal and appendiceal cancer. World J Surg 19:235-240, 1995.
6. Conte CC, Petrelli NJ, Stulc J, et al: Adenocarcinoma of the appendix. Surg Gynecol Obstet 166:451-453, 1988.
7. Andersson A, Bergdahl L, Boquist L: Primary carcinoma of the appendix. Ann Surg 183:53-57, 1976.

David Feltquate, MD, PhD

PATIENT 61

A 67-year-old man with a rising prostate-specific antigen level

A 67-year-old man presents with a rising serum prostate specific antigen (PSA) level. His past medical history is notable for prostate adenocarcinoma. He was originally diagnosed 2 years prior, when he was found on routine screening to have an elevated PSA (8.1) and an abnormal digital rectal exam. Following a transrectal prostrate biopsy that showed a Gleason 7 prostrate adenocarcinoma, he underwent a radical retropubic prostatectomy, which revealed a Gleason 7 (4+3) tumor with extracapsular extension but no seminal vesicle invasion, negative margins, and no tumor involvement in sampled pelvic lymph nodes. Within 2 months following surgery, his PSA became undetectable and remained undetectable for 15 months. However, it has risen over the last 6 months with a doubling time of 3 months. On review of symptoms, he denies any urinary or musculoskeletal complaints.

Physical Examination: General: well-appearing, no acute distress. Vital signs: normal. HEENT: anicteric, clear oropharynx. Lymph nodes: no lymphadenopathy. Chest: clear to auscultation. Cardiac: regular rate and rhythm, without murmurs. Abdomen: soft, nontender, no hepatosplenomegaly. Musculoskeletal: no spinal tenderness. Extremities: no edema. Rectal exam: prostatic fossa without masses or nodularity.

Laboratory Findings: CBC, renal function, and liver function tests: normal. PSA values are noted chronologically (see Table). Bone scan: no evidence of osseous metastases. CT scan of abdomen and pelvis: surgical staples in pelvis, no masses or pelvic lymphadenopathy.

PSA Values in Relation to the Timing of Radical Retropubic Prostatectomy (RRP)

	Pre-RRP	2 mo	6 mo	9 mo	12 mo	15 mo	18 mo	21 mo	24 mo
PSA	8.1	< 0.05	< 0.05	< 0.05	< 0.05	< 0.05	.23	.45	.93

mo = month; PSA = prostate specific antigen.

Question: What are the management options for the patient's biochemical relapse?

Answer: Multiple initial management strategies exist, including: observation with close clinical follow up; first-line hormonal therapy/androgen depleting strategies (surgical or pharmaceutical); intermittent androgen deprivation; salvage radiotherapy; or enrollment in a clinical trial. Specific disease characteristics can be used to predict the likelihood of progression, to stratify risk, and to guide management. In this patient, although observation or enrollment in a clinical trial are acceptable initial strategies, based on his PSA doubling time, his risk of developing overt metastatic disease is high enough to consider first-line hormonal therapy in the near future.

Discussion: Prostate cancer is the most common noncutaneous malignancy in men, with approximately 220,000 cases diagnosed annually. Treatment for localized disease includes radical prostatectomy and radiotherapy. A substantial fraction of these patients will experience recurrence; in many patients, a rising PSA will be the initial indicator of this disease state.

The kinetics of PSA measurement vary with the type of treatment. PSA has a serum half-life of approximately 3 days. Thus, within weeks after a radical retropubic prostatectomy (RRP), the PSA should be undetectable. Following radiotherapy, the PSA decline does not follow single-order decay kinetics and may reach a nadir as long as 12 to 24 months after therapy. Although this nadir may be measurable in radiotherapy-treated patients, it should reach a relatively stable plateau. A rising PSA from a measurable baseline is considered to be evidence of disease progression.

Causes of a rising PSA after primary therapy include one of the following three situations: local recurrence, metastatic disease, or a combination of both. Factors that favor metastatic recurrence include high Gleason grade, rapid PSA doubling time, capsular penetration, seminal vesicle invasion, or rapid post-surgical biochemical relapse. Determining whether a patient has local or metastatic disease can be difficult. Despite the use of studies, such as bone scan, abdominal and pelvic CT scan, and/or pelvic MRI with endorectal probe, many patients do not have radiographically detectable disease.

Although biochemical relapse signifies disease progression, whether this is clinically meaningful is less certain. Several studies have reported that the rate of development of overt metastatic disease varies from patient to patient. For prostatectomy patients, factors that portend a more aggressive course of disease include PSA doubling time (< 10 months), time to biochemical relapse (< 2 years), and Gleason pathological score (≥ 8). Recent evidence suggests that a doubling time of less than 6 months predicts the development of bone lesions within 1 year, and an annual PSA velocity of greater than 2.0 ng/mL is associated with a significantly shorter time to death.

Based on a patient's risk for development of metastases in the context of life expectancy (without cancer), a decision to treat can be made. The optimal time to begin treatment is controversial. There have been no studies showing a survival benefit for early hormone therapy treatment. Early treatment, however, may delay time to overt disease progression. Thus, there is no threshold PSA value at which treatment should begin.

Numerous initial management strategies exist, including:

- Observation with close clinical follow-up.
- First-line hormonal therapy/androgen depleting strategies (including surgical castration or medical castration with an LHRH-agonist with or without an androgen receptor blocker).
- Intermittent androgen deprivation (associated with improved quality of life compared to continuous androgen deprivation).
- Salvage radiotherapy or salvage prostatectomy.
- Enrollment in a clinical trial testing new therapies.

Factors correlating with a successful outcome following salvage radiotherapy include Gleason score (≤ 7), pre-XRT PSA (< 2.0), positive surgical margins, and PSA doubling time (> 10 months).

The present patient had a Gleason 7 adenocarcinoma and a rising PSA 18 months after his RRP. His biochemical relapse signified disease progression. Serial measurements of his PSA demonstrated a doubling time of 3 months. Using the Pound prediction tables, he was found to have a 77% likelihood of remaining metastases-free at 3 years, a 42% likelihood at 5 years, and a 24% likelihood at 7 years *without* any treatment. For salvage XRT, he has only a 22% chance of progression-free survival at 4 years. Although close observation or enrollment in a clinical trial are acceptable strategies for this patient, based on his PSA doubling time, his risk for the development of overt metastatic disease is high enough to consider beginning first-line hormonal therapy in the near future.

Clinical Pearls

1. A rising PSA after primary therapy signifies local recurrence, metastatic disease, or a combination of both.

2. The optimal management for biochemical relapse is controversial, with several possible strategies.

3. Prediction models may be used to risk-stratify patients and guide management decisions.

REFERENCES

1. D'Amico AV, Chen MH, Roehl KA, Catalona WJ: Preoperative PSA velocity and the risk of death from prostate cancer after radical prostatectomy. N Engl J Med 351(2):125-135, 2004.
2. Stephenson AJ, Shariat SF, Zelefsky MJ: Salvage radiotherapy for recurrent prostate cancer after radical prostatectomy. JAMA 291:1325, 2004.
3. Pound CR, Partin AW, Eisenberger MA: Natural history of progression after PSA elevation following radical prostatectomy. JAMA 281:1591, 1999.
4. Carroll PR, Lee KL, Fuks ZY, Kantoff PW: Cancer of the prostate. In (ed): Cancer: Principles and Practice of Oncology, 6th ed.

PATIENT 62

A 46-year-old woman with abdominal bloating and vaginal bleeding

A 46-year-old woman with no significant medical history presents to her physician with a 2-month history of abdominal bloating, constipation, and vaginal bleeding. Her review of systems is positive for 17-pound weight loss and increasing fatigue. She is G2P2 and had her first child at age 32. She denies a history of oral contraceptive use. Her last menstrual period was 3 months ago. The patient has a seven-pack-year smoking history but quit several years ago. She has had normal mammography and colonoscopy results within the past year. There is no family history of malignancy.

Physical Examination: Temperature 36.2°C, blood pressure 118/65 mmHg, pulse 88. General: fatigued appearance. HEENT: anicteric sclerae, oropharynx clear, no adenopathy. Cardiovascular: regular rate and rhythm, without murmurs. Chest: clear to auscultation. Breasts: no palpable masses, skin changes, or nipple discharge. Abdomen: soft, large pelvic mass extending from pelvis into abdomen, with mild right lower quadrant (RLQ) tenderness to palpation; no rebound or guarding. Extremities: no clubbing, cyanosis, or edema. Skin: no ecchymoses, petechiae, or rashes. Pelvis: difficult to delineate, large pelvic mass extending to the level of the umbilicus, normal cervix, old blood in the vaginal vault, no vulvar or vaginal lesions.

Laboratory Findings: Hemoglobin 10.3 g/dL, platelets: 290,000/μL, WBC 5200/μL. Basic metabolic profile: normal. CA125: 691. CEA: 20.6. CA19-9: 120. Pelvic ultrasound: 14-cm pelvic mass and fibroid uterus. CT scan of abdomen and pelvis with contrast: 14 cm × 13.4 cm multi-loculated pelvic mass abutting the bladder with peritoneal soft tissue thickening (see Figure). Chest radiograph: normal. Pap smear cytology: atypical cells suspicious for carcinoma.

Questions: What is the most likely diagnosis? What is the appropriate surgical approach to this disease? Is there a role for adjuvant therapy?

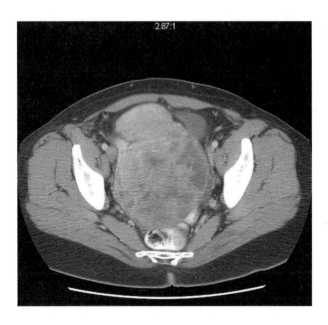

Answers: Ovarian cancer is the most likely diagnosis. The surgical approach should include total abdominal hysterectomy and bilateral salpingo-oophorectomy. Yes, there is a role for adjuvant therapy.

Discussion: Ovarian cancer accounts for nearly 30% of all gynecological malignancies (approximately 23,000 cases per year) and represents over 14,000 deaths annually (53% of gynecological cancer deaths). While early-stage ovarian cancer has 5-year survival rates as high as 80%, advanced ovarian cancer survival rates range from 5 to 30%. Unfortunately, more than 75% of patients present with advanced disease because early malignancy is typically asymptomatic. When symptoms do occur, they are usually nonspecific, such as irregular menses, abdominal discomfort or distention, constipation, or urinary frequency. Although physical examination, CA125, and imaging techniques may be useful in assessing response to therapy, they have not proven useful as screening modalities for ovarian cancer in the general population.

The diagnosis of ovarian cancer is made by pathological evaluation following exploratory laparotomy. In fact, the staging system (see Table) for ovarian cancer, developed by the International Federation of Gynecology and Obstetrics, is based upon the results of a thorough and appropriate operation. This surgery should include total abdominal hysterectomy and bilateral salpingo-oophorectomy, tumor debulking, examination of all visceral and parietal surfaces within the peritoneal cavity, omentectomy, diaphragmatic sampling, and selective pelvic and para-aortic node sampling. Reproductive organ conservation is an option for fertile women with stage IA disease (limited to one ovary); this spares the uterus and contralateral ovary and fallopian tube.

The critical first step in the management of ovarian cancer is optimal *cytoreductive surgery* or *debulking.* Optimal debulking is defined as cumulative postoperative residual disease less than or equal to 1 cm. Griffiths and colleagues reported that thorough debulking led to improved survival rates, with 0 cm and greater than 1.5 cm residual disease yielding overall survival of 39 and 11 months, respectively. Recent data support a survival advantage to primary optimal debulking as well as to interval debulking after chemotherapy for those patients with initially unresectable disease.

Ten percent to 50% of patients who undergo optimal debulking will have recurrence of their disease. Stages IA and IB well-differentiated tumors have excellent survival rates (5-year survival 90-98%); however, the presence of high-risk features, such as moderate to poor differentiation, stage IC disease, stage II disease, or clear-cell histology, identifies a population that may benefit from the addition of *chemotherapy.* Several randomized trials have supported post-surgical chemotherapy with paclitaxel and a platinum-based regimen.

The Italian Inter-Regional Cooperative Group performed two randomized trials comparing platinum-based chemotherapy to (1) observation or (2) intraperitoneal P_{32}. There was no significant difference in 5-year overall survival between

International Federation of Gynecology and Obstetrics Staging System

	Stage I: Tumor Limited to the Ovaries
IA	Limited to one ovary
IB	Bilateral ovaries involved
IC	One or both ovaries involved, capsular rupture, positive cytology on washings, tumor on ovarian surface

	Stage II: Pelvic Extension and/or Implants
IIA	Extension of disease or metastasis to uterus and/or fallopian tubes
IIB	Extension of disease or metastasis to other pelvic organs
IIC	Either IIA or IIB with capsular rupture, positive cytology on washings, tumor on ovarian surface

	Stage III: Peritoneal Implants Outside of the Pelvis or Positive Lymph Nodes
IIIA	Microscopic seeding of abdominal peritoneal surfaces
IIIB	Abdominal peritoneal implants < 2 cm in diameter
IIIC	Abdominal peritoneal implants > 2 cm in diameter and/or positive retroperitoneal or inguinal lymph nodes

	Stage IV: Metastatic Parenchymal Disease

arms; however, systemic therapy was better tolerated by patients. A Scandinavian study randomized patients with early-stage ovarian cancer to either observation or postoperative cisplatin. In this study, there was no difference in disease-free survival or disease-specific survival. Unfortunately, both of these trials lacked power and did not take into consideration the extent of cytoreduction.

Large cooperative group trials (GOG-111 and OV-10) demonstrated a significant survival advantage to platinum-based therapy together with paclitaxel as compared to cyclophosphamide. The GOG 158 and AGO-OVAR3 trials both demonstrated no difference in response rate when carboplatin was compared with cisplatin. The EORTC-ACTION trial found an improvement in disease-free survival with adjuvant chemotherapy. The ICON1 trial demonstrated a 7% improvement in 5-year overall survival in patients with early-stage ovarian cancer receiving adjuvant chemotherapy compared with women treated at the time of relapse (75% vs 82%). These data have led to the *current standard of care* for adjuvant therapy in *early-stage epithelial ovarian cancer*: paclitaxel 175 mg/m^2 and carboplatin AUC 5-7.5 for three to six cycles.

The present patient had limited-stage epithelial ovarian cancer; her atypical symptom of vaginal bleeding prompted her to seek medical attention. Surgical pathology from this patient's resection revealed high-grade mixed endometrioid and serous adenocarcinoma of the bilateral ovaries. Lymphovascular invasion was present. Biopsy of the omentum was free of malignant cells, although a biopsy of the cul-de-sac revealed adenocarcinoma. Cytology from pelvic washings was positive for malignant cells. None of the 45 lymph nodes sampled were involved with tumor. Her disease was stage IIC. She underwent chemotherapy comprising of carboplatin and paclitaxel.

Clinical Pearls

1. Epithelial ovarian cancer is rarely diagnosed at an early stage because there are few symptoms when disease is localized to the ovary.

2. Diagnosis and accurate staging require optimal cytoreduction, including total abdominal hysterectomy and bilateral salpingo-oophorectomy, examination of all visceral and parietal surfaces within the peritoneal cavity, tumor debulking, omentectomy, diaphragmatic sampling, and selective pelvic and para-aortic node sampling.

3. Adjuvant chemotherapy with paclitaxel 175 mg/m^2 and carboplatin AUC 5-7.5 is the standard of care for patients with disease beyond stage IA/B, grade 1 or grade 2.

REFERENCES

1. Bookman MA, Greer BE, Ozols RF: Optimal therapy of advanced ovarian cancer: Carboplatin and paclitaxel vs. cisplatin and paclitaxel (GOG 158) and an update on GOG0 182-ICON5. Int J Gynecol Cancer 13:735-740, 2003.
2. Goff BA, Mandel L, Muntz HG, Melancon CH: Ovarian carcinoma diagnosis. Cancer 89(10):2068-2075, 2000.
3. Piccart MJ, Bertelsen K, James K, et al: Randomized Intergroup Trial of Cisplatin-Paclitaxel versus Cisplatin-Cyclophosphamide in women with advanced epithelial ovarian cancer: Three year results. J Natl Cancer Inst 92:699-708, 2000.
4. Trope C, Kaern J, Hogberg T, et al: Randomized study on adjuvant chemotherapy in stage I high-risk ovarian cancer with evaluation of DNA-ploidy as prognostic instrument. Ann Oncol 11:281-288, 2000.
5. Dubois A, Lueck HJ, Meier W: Cisplatin/paclitaxel vs. carboplatin/paclitaxel in ovarian cancer. Update of am Arbeitsgemeinschaft Gynakologie (AGO) Study Group Trial. Proc ASCO 18:A1374, 1999.
6. McGuire WP, Hoskins WJ, Brady MF, et al: Cyclophosphamide and cisplatin compared with paclitaxel and cisplatin in patients with stage III and stage IV ovarian cancer. New Engl J Med 334:1-6, 1996.
7. Bolis G, Colombo N, Pecorelli S, et al: Adjuvant treatment for early epithelial ovarian cancer: Results of two randomized clinical trials comparing cisplatin to no further treatment or chromic phosphate. GICOG. Ann Oncol 6:887-893, 1995.
8. Griffiths CT: Surgical resection of tumor bulk in the primary treatment of ovarian carcinoma. Natl Cancer Inst Monogr 42:101-104, 1975.

David Feltquate, MD, PhD

PATIENT 63

A 61-year-old man with lower extremity edema

A 61-year-old man complains of new lower extremity edema. His past medical history is notable for prostate cancer. He was originally diagnosed with a Gleason 8 (4 + 4) prostate adenocarcinoma 7 years prior, following a workup for elevated prostate specific antigen (PSA). His localized disease was treated with external beam radiation therapy (EBRT), and his PSA reached a nadir of 1.2 within 15 months of treatment. Five years ago a biochemical relapse developed, and 4 years ago hormonal therapy with leuprolide was initiated. His PSA remained undetectable until 1 year ago, at which time he experienced a short-lived response to flutamide but no response to flutamide-withdrawal or to keto-conazole. Over the past month, bilateral lower extremity edema has developed. On review of symptoms, he describes recent onset of nocturia and hesitancy, as well as left-sided hip pain.

Physical Examination: General: well-appearing, no acute distress. Vital signs: normal. HEENT: anicteric, clear oropharynx. Chest: clear to auscultation. Cardiac: regular rate and rhythm, without murmurs. Abdomen: soft, nontender, no hepatosplenomegaly. Musculoskeletal: no spinal tenderness. Extremities: bilateral 2+ pitting edema to knees. Rectal exam: 35-g prostate without nodularity or masses.

Laboratory Findings: CBC and liver function tests: normal. BUN 16, creatinine 0.9. PSA 17.3, testosterone < 12. Bilateral lower extremity Doppler ultrasound: no evidence of deep-venous thrombosis. CT scan of abdomen and pelvis: bulky pelvic lymphadenopathy with left-sided hydroureter but no hydronephrosis. Bone scan: new metastases in the left ischium, T_{10} vertebrae, and several ribs, bilaterally.

Question: What is the recommended treatment for this patient?

Answer: The recommended treatment for metastatic androgen-independent prostate cancer is a docetaxel-containing chemotherapy regimen. Palliative radiation to sites of painful lesions, nephrostomy tube placement, and/or zoledronic acid may also be considered.

Discussion: Androgen-independent prostate cancer is difficult to treat. Historically, prostate cancer was not found to be especially chemosensitive, with response rates in the 10 to 20% range. During the past decade, however, newer agents and combination regimens have significantly improved the treatment armamentarium. Prior to 2004 there was no gold standard, although a combination of mitoxantrone and prednisone was FDA-approved based on palliative properties (quality of life scores, pain relief) rather than due to survival benefit, PSA decline, or tumor size response rates. But the standard of care for treatment of metastatic androgen-independent prostate cancer has changed. Two independent phase III studies have demonstrated that docetaxel-containing regimens yield a survival advantage over mitoxantrone/prednisone (used as a historical "standard"). In one trial, docetaxel and estramustine given every 3 weeks was associated with a 23% improvement in survival. In a second trial, docetaxel and prednisone administered every 3 weeks led to a similarly enhanced survival. The median absolute increase in survival was 3 to 3.5 months.

The most active agents in prostate cancer appear to be drugs that disrupt microtubule function. The taxanes, vinca alkaloids, and estramustine all possess low-level single-agent activity. Some combination regimens with these agents appear to have synergistic activity with response rates exceeding 50%. Other drugs, such as doxorubicin, cyclophosphamide, carboplatin, and etoposide, have little single-agent activity but improve efficacy when used in combination with microtubule-disrupting drugs. However, significant toxicity can result, limiting their utility. For example, combinations with estramustine increase the thromboembolic event rate up to 10 to 20%, necessitating the use of prophylactic low-dose anticoagulation during treatment.

Involved field radiotherapy (IFRT) to symptomatic sites of disease serves as an important mode of treatment. Indications include: poorly controlled pain due to bony metastases, risk for epidural disease, and mechanical obstruction due to bulky disease.

The present patient had symptomatic bulky pelvic lymphadenopathy and new bony metastases. He was at risk for developing left-sided hydronephrosis. He was started on a docetaxel-containing regimen with estramustine. His radiation oncologist was consulted to determine whether he was a candidate for palliative IFRT to his left pelvic lymph nodes to avert left hydronephrosis (he may not have been suitable based on his prior treatment field, because radiation to a previously irradiated area can result in significant toxicity). If his pelvic lymph nodes do not respond to therapy, his urologist will be consulted to consider placement of a nephrostomy tube. Use of the bisphosphonate, zoledronic acid, may help reduce skeletal complications from bony metastases (assuming renal function is normal). Should the patient's disease progress, treatment with other agents (monotherapy or in combination) or enrollment in a clinical trial can be considered.

Clinical Pearls

1. The standard of care for treatment of metastatic androgen-independent prostate cancer includes a docetaxel-containing regimen.
2. Palliative radiation therapy can be considered for management of metastatic sites.
3. Zoledronic acid may reduce skeletal complications due to bony metastases.

REFERENCES

1. Tannock IF: Docetaxel plus prednisone or mitoxantrone plus prednisone for advanced prostrate cancer. N Engl J Med 351:1502-1512, 2004.
2. Petrylak DP: Docetaxel and estramustine compared with mitoxantrone and prednisone for advanced refractory prostrate cancer. N Engl J Med 351:1513-1520, 2004.

PATIENT 64

A 42-year-old man with a new right-sided flank mass

A 42-year-old man presents to clinic with a growing palpable nodule in his right flank. His past medical history is notable for a right laparoscopic nephrectomy 2 years prior for renal cell carcinoma, which was 6 cm in diameter and did not invade the capsule. There was no evidence of disease outside the kidney at that time. The patient was without complaint until 3 months ago, when right upper quadrant discomfort and back pain developed. More recently, he noted a growing palpable nodule in his right flank. He denies fevers, chills, weight loss, and hematuria.

Physical Examination: General: well-appearing, no apparent distress. Vital signs: temperature 37.2°C, blood pressure 114/70 mmHg, pulse 80, respirations 16, weight 78 kg. HEENT: sclera anicteric, oropharynx clear. Chest: clear to auscultation. Cardiac: normal S_1, S_2; no murmurs, rubs, or gallops. Abdomen: soft, nontender, nondistended, no palpable organomegaly. Back: 3 cm × 4 cm fixed nodular mass palpable in right flank. Skin: no rash.

Laboratory Findings: Extended chemistry panel: normal. CT scan of abdomen and pelvis: multiple nodular masses, including a 5-cm bilobed mass involving right nephrectomy surgical bed, mass adjacent to peritoneal cavity on right, and mass at incision site. PET scan: increased FDG uptake the right flank, right adrenal region, right renal fossa bed, and posterior abdominal wall.

Question: What is the diagnosis?

Diagnosis: The patient has recurrent renal cell carcinoma.

Discussion: There are approximately 30,000 cases of renal cell carcinoma per year in the United States. Over 40% of these patients have metastatic disease at diagnosis. Therefore, at the time of diagnosis, patients are imaged to evaluate for distant metastases or disease beyond the renal capsule. Surgical therapy is generally recommended for patients with early-stage disease who can be cured by the procedure. Radical nephrectomy or laparoscopic nephrectomy are both acceptable options, with no difference seen in overall survival.

The median survival for patients with metastatic disease is less than 1 year. Fewer than 10% of patients with metastatic disease are alive at 10 years. In patients with metastatic disease, *five prognostic factors* have been found to aid in predicting survival:

1. Low Karnofsky performance status (less than 80%).
2. Elevated lactic dehydrogenase.
3. Low hemoglobin (less than 10).
4. High corrected serum calcium (greater than 10).
5. Absence of prior nephrectomy.

Nephrectomy has also been shown to benefit patients who present initially with metastatic disease. Patients with recurrent disease who can undergo a metastasectomy have better survival rates. The fewer number of metastatic sites predicts better survival. Cytotoxic chemotherapy and hormonal therapy have been found to be effective less than 10% of the time in metastatic disease. Radiation therapy is generally only beneficial in metastatic disease for palliation of brain metastases or symptomatic bony disease.

Immunotherapy has been the focus of numerous studies in metastatic renal cell carcinoma. Interferon-α has been found to produce a response in approximately 14 to 17% of patients and an improvement in median survival of 2.5 months. If a patient responds to interferon, the response duration is usually 4 to 6 months. This mild benefit must be weighed against the toxicity of the drug. Interferon-α commonly causes a flu-like syndrome throughout treatment. Other common adverse effects include depression, nausea, diarrhea, liver dysfunction, and myelosuppression. A standard regimen involves subcutaneous injections three times a week. Pegylated interferon, which allows less frequent dosing, is under evaluation as a potential treatment.

Interleukin-2 (IL-2) has shown a response rate of approximately 15% in metastatic renal cell cancer. The high-dose regimen of IL-2 uses 600,000 to 720,000 units/kg every 8 hours for 5 days and often requires an ICU admission. A small number of patients treated with high-dose IL-2 have been found to have a complete response of prolonged duration. This must be tempered with the toxicity profile; interleukin-2 can produce severe side effects, including hemodynamic instability, pulmonary edema, arrhythmias, capillary leak syndrome, and death. Low-dose IL-2 is also being evaluated. A recent study found no difference in overall survival between low-dose and high-dose intravenous IL-2.

Combination therapy with interferon and interleukin-2 has been evaluated. In one trial comparing combination treatment to monotherapy with interferon-α, no benefit for combination therapy was found. Treatment with interferon-α or IL-2 is better tolerated in patients with high performance status. If either cytokine is chosen, patients should receive treatment at a center experienced with their administration. Patients should be monitored with serial imaging.

Allogeneic transplant has been evaluated for metastatic renal cell carcinoma and has produced a small number of complete remissions. The mortality of this procedure makes it a less desirable option. Trials are underway studying the role of anti-angiogenesis agents in this disease; at ASCO in 2004, one trial found a 30% response rate in metastatic RCC patients.

The present patient had initially renal cell cancer staged as T_{1b}, N_x, M_0 (his lymph nodes were not assessed). He now has recurrent disease with multiple sites of metastases, making surgery an ineffective option. The patient is considering treatment with interferon or a clinical trial.

Clinical Pearls

1. Surgical treatment is recommended for patients with potentially curable renal cell carcinoma, or for selected metastasectomies.

2. Standard cytotoxic chemotherapy, hormonal therapy, or radiation therapy has not been shown to improve survival in patients with metastatic disease.

3. Interferon-α and interleukin-2 have demonstrated modest responses in metastatic renal cell carcinoma.

REFERENCES

1. Motzer RJ, Rini BI, Michaelson MD, et al: SU011248, a novel tyrosine kinase inhibitor, shows antitumor activity in second-line therapy for patients with metastatic renal cell carcinoma: Results of a phase 2 trial. ASCO Proceedings 22(14S):4500, 2004.
2. Martel CL, Lara PN: Renal cell carcinoma: Current status and future directions. Crit Rev Oncol Hematol 45:177-190, 2003.
3. Yang JC, Sherry RM, Steinberg SM, et al: Randomized study of high-dose and low-dose interleukin-2 in patients with metastatic renal cancer. J Clin Oncol 21(16):3127-3132, 2003.
4. Flanigan RC, Salmon SE, Blumenstein BA, et al: Nephrectomy followed by interferon alfa-2b compared with interferon alfa-2b alone for metastatic renal-cell cancer. N Engl J Med 345:1655-1659, 2001.
5. Motzer RJ, Mazumdar M, Bacik J, et al: Survival and prognostic stratification of 670 patients with advanced renal cell carcinoma. J Clin Oncol 17(8):2530-2537, 1999.
6. Motzer RJ, Bander NH, Nanus DM: Renal-cell carcinoma. N Engl J Med 335(12):865-875, 1996.
7. Atkins MB, Sparano J, Fisher RI, et al: Randomized phase II trial of high-dose interleukin-2 either alone or in combination with interferon alfa-2b in advanced renal cell carcinoma. J Clin Oncol 11(4):661-670, 1993.

Igor Matushansky, MD

PATIENT 65

A 54-year-old woman with increasing pigmentation of a preexisting mole

A 54-year-old woman without any significant medical history has a pigmented lesion, which had recently become darker, excised from her mid back for cosmetic reasons. Pathology identifies it to be melanoma with a depth of 1.5 mm. She has a wide local excision and sentinel lymph node mapping leading to the discovery of one sentinel lymph node that stains positive for melanoma in the right axilla. A complete dissection of the right axilla reveals no other lymph nodes involved. CT scans of the head, chest, abdomen, and pelvis indicate no evidence of metastatic disease.

Physical Examination: Temperature 37°C, blood pressure 110/80 mmHg, pulse 76. General: well appearing, no acute distress. HEENT: mild pallor, anicteric, no adenopathy. Cardiovascular: regular rate and rhythm, without murmurs. Chest: clear to auscultation. Abdomen: nontender, nondistended, no hepatosplenomegaly. Extremities: no cyanosis, clubbing, or edema. Skin: no rashes, no purpura, no petechiae; well-healing surgical scars on mid back and right axilla. No other atypical lesions noted.

Laboratory Findings: Hemoglobin 12.5 g/dL, platelets 292,000/μL, WBC 8200/μL (normal differential). Biochemistry profile (including LDH): normal. Liver function tests: normal.

Questions: What is the patient's stage? What is the appropriate treatment?

Answers: This patient has stage IIIA melanoma. Interferon is the only FDA-approved therapy in the adjuvant treatment of malignant melanoma; however, its use is associated with significant toxicity and marginal benefit.

Discussion: Currently, patients with local disease are usually treated surgically with wide excision (defined as 1 cm margin for 1 mm depth of the primary) followed by sentinel lymph node mapping (only if the primary is greater than 1 mm deep or Clark level IV/V). Assuming the sentinel lymph node does not show evidence of melanoma, no further treatment is recommended because the chance of recurrence is fairly low. On the other extreme, patients with metastatic disease are usually treated with single-agent dacarbazine (DTIC) or a DTIC-based regimen with variable response rates.

However, the question of how to treat those patients who have locally advanced and/or lymph node–positive disease remains unanswered. This subset of patients has an extremely variable relapse rate (20-75% over 5 years following diagnosis), which can be estimated based on the size of the primary and the number of involved lymph nodes on presentation. Historically, multiple chemotherapy agents have been examined in the adjuvant setting and were found to have no benefit. The only agent that has shown any activity in the adjuvant setting is high-dose interferon (20 megaunits [MU]/m^2 IV daily M–F $\times$ 4 weeks; then 10 MU/m^2 subcutaneously TIW $\times$ 48 weeks), and currently it is the only FDA-approved treatment for locally advanced and/or lymph node (LN)-positive (resected) melanoma.

The evidence for interferon comes from several Eastern Cooperative Oncology Group (ECOG) trials performed in the late 1990s. ECOG 1684 enrolled patients with locally advanced and/or LN-positive (nonmetastatic) melanoma and randomized them to high-dose interferon (IFN) versus observation. Initial results demonstrated a 9% overall survival advantage for high-dose IFN with a 1-year delay in time to recurrence; however, the significance of the survival advantage has been lost with additional follow-up. ECOG 1690 similarly compared high-dose IFN, low-dose IFN, and observation. The data showed a relapse-free survival advantage but no overall survival advantage. Finally, ECOG 1694 compared high-dose IFN to the GMK ganglioside vaccine. This study demonstrated an advantage in relapse-free survival and overall survival for the interferon arm over vaccine therapy. High-dose IFN is associated with significant toxicities ranging from flu-like symptoms to clinical depression. Supportive medications (including selective serotonin receptor inhibitors [SSRIs]) have been implemented to lessen these effects as more experience is gained with the drug.

In summary, although studies may demonstrate that high-dose IFN has some efficacy in the adjuvant treatment of locally advanced and/or LN-positive melanoma, its significant side effect profile (extreme fatigue, hepatotoxicity, myelosuppression, neuropsychiatric) as well as difficult administration profile (IV/SQ, every other day for 1 year) usually lead to an involved pro/con discussion between the patient and the oncologist. Thus, although interferon remains the only FDA-approved treatment for locally advanced and/or LN-positive melanoma, it is difficult to categorize it as the "standard of care." Alternatives for adjuvant therapy currently being employed run the gamut from various immune system modifiers (e.g., vaccines, cytokines) to observation alone.

After a prolonged discussion in which the previous data were presented to the patient, she decided to receive *low*-dose IFN therapy (which does not have the side effect profile of high-dose IFN) for 6 months. The patient tolerated the treatment well and, afterward, was enrolled on a dendritic cell vaccine protocol. She completed the protocol without any adverse events. She is currently off all treatments and remains without evidence of recurrence 2.5 years later. Whether her current disease-free status is a result of her treatment choices or the fact that her chance of recurrence was relatively low (25%, given that she began with a shallow primary and a micrometastases in one sentinel LN) will not be known until more data regarding the mechanism of action of interferon, the efficacy of vaccines, and the biology of melanoma become better known.

Clinical Pearls

1. Patients with local disease are usually treated surgically with wide excision (defined as 1 cm margin for 1 mm depth of the primary) followed by sentinel lymph node mapping (only if the primary is greater than 1 mm deep or Clark level IV/V).

2. The only agent that has shown any activity in the adjuvant setting is high-dose interferon (20 MU/m^2 IV daily M–F × 4 weeks; then 10 MU/m^2 subcutaneously TIW × 48 weeks), and, currently, it is the only FDA-approved treatment for locally advanced and/or LN-positive (resected) melanoma.

3. High-dose interferon treatment is associated with significant toxicity.

REFERENCES

1. National Comprehensive Cancer Network: Clinical Practice Guidelines in Oncology, 2004. http://www.nccn.org/professionals/physician_gls/default.asp

2. Kirkwood JM, Ibrahim JG, Sosman JA, et al: High-dose interferon alfa-2b significantly prolongs relapse-free and overall survival compared with the GM2-KLH/QS-21 vaccine in patients with resected stage IIB-III melanoma. Results of Intergroup Trial E1694/S9512/C509801. J Clin Oncol 19:2370-2380, 2001.

3. Kirkwood JM, Ibrahim JG, Sondak VK, et al: High- and low-dose interferon alfa-2b in high-risk melanoma: First analysis of intergroup trial E1690/S9111/C9190. J Clin Oncol 18:2444-2458, 2000.

4. Kirkwood JM, Strawderman MH, Ernstoff MS, et al: Interferon alfa-2b adjuvant therapy of high-risk resected cutaneous melanoma: The Eastern Cooperative Oncology Group Trial EST 1684. J Clin Oncol 18:2444-2458, 2000.

PATIENT 66

A 55-year-old man with abdominal pain and a history of cutaneous and ocular melanoma

A 55-year-old man presents with right upper quadrant abdominal pain. Past medical history is significant for cutaneous melanoma of the left scapula, status post wide excision and negative sentinel lymph node biopsy, and ocular melanoma, for which the patient underwent enucleation. He has a strong family history of cutaneous melanoma.

Physical Examination: Temperature 37.8°C, pulse 80, blood pressure 165/92 mmHg. General: no acute distress. HEENT: left glass eye, right eye mildly icteric. Cardiovascular: regular rate and rhythm, without murmurs. Chest: decreased breath sounds bibasilar. Abdomen: obese, liver palpable 4 cm below costal margin. Extremities: no peripheral edema. Skin: fair, well-healed scar left scapula, no suspicious lesions.

Laboratory Findings: WBC 10,000/μL, hemoglobin 13.3 g/dL, platelets 286,000/μL. Biochemistry profile: electrolytes normal. BUN 12, creatinine 0.8. Liver function tests: AST 86, ALT 81, alkaline phosphatase 349, total bilirubin 0.8, total protein 8.1, albumin 3.5, LDH 1064. CT scans of chest, abdomen, and pelvis: diffuse hepatic metastases (see Figure).

Questions: What is the most likely cause of the patient's lab abnormalities? Which diagnostic tests should be ordered?

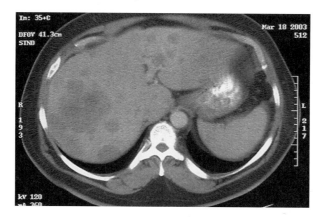

Answers: Metastatic ocular melanoma is the likely cause of the lab abnormalities. A liver biopsy is the diagnostic test to order, at this point.

Discussion: Ocular melanoma is a rare malignancy that threatens both sight and life and is the only potentially fatal ocular malignancy in adults. In the white population it has an average annual incidence of 6 cases per million, with approximately 1200 cases diagnosed each year. White men have 72 times the risk of developing ocular melanoma compared to African American men. There is a higher incidence in older men, who probably have higher sun exposure, than in older women and in residents of rural areas, where outdoor work is more prevalent. The incidence in dark-eyed populations is low, and the preferential location of ocular melanoma is in ocular sites known to receive the highest exposure to solar radiation. Protective factors are olive or black skin, brown iris color, wearing prescription glasses, and high resistance to sunburn. Ocular melanomas are the most common primary intraocular malignancy in whites.

The annual age-adjusted incidence of ocular melanoma is one-eighth that of cutaneous melanoma in the United States. The observed increase in incidence of cutaneous melanomas has not been observed for ocular melanomas. Although a relationship between primary ocular melanoma and cutaneous melanoma has been proposed, there are no guidelines about whether patients diagnosed with ocular melanoma should have dermatological examinations or, conversely, whether those with cutaneous melanoma should have ophthalmological evaluations.

As in cutaneous disease, early recognition and diagnosis of ocular melanoma is essential, because therapeutic intervention can be curative in the early stages only. Until radiation therapy gained wide acceptance, enucleation was the standard treatment for ocular melanoma. Recently, radiotherapy with radioactive plaques sutured to sclera is gaining favor as the standard therapy. The survival rates are similar, but the eye is preserved, frequently with useful vision. Other treatment options are radiation therapy, photocoagulation, transpupillary thermotherapy, photochemotherapy, and local resection. Enucleation should be considered in only patients with large tumors, large extrascleral extension, or neovascular glaucoma. Small tumors (<10 mm in diameter and 2 mm in height) are often observed in asymptomatic patients until growth is documented. Ocular melanomas have a purely hematogenous pattern of dissemination, with involvement of the liver in 90% of cases. There is no lymphangitic spread due to absence of lymphatics in the eye.

Patients should be followed with physical exams, chest X-ray, and liver function tests. However, regular monitoring might be considered of limited benefit, given the limited impact of treatment in patients with metastatic disease.

Poor prognostic factors include large tumor size, tumor involvement of the ciliary body, increased age, and extracapsular extension. Median survival for patients with metastatic disease is 2 to 9 months. Despite advances in achieving local control, 50% of patients die eventually of distant metastases. Most commonly there is hematogenous dissemination to the liver. Metastases to other sites (lung, bone, heart, GI tract, lymph nodes, pancreas, skin) occur generally in association with liver metastasis. Performance status, largest dimension of the largest metastasis, and serum alkaline phosphatase significantly correlate with survival.

Surgical resection of solitary metastasis provides long-term survival in rare cases only. The response rates to chemotherapy are disappointing, but regional therapy with isolated hepatic perfusion chemotherapy has shown promising results. Single-institution studies on hepatic chemoembolization and intra-arterial fotemustine- and platinum-based chemotherapy for hepatic metastases now report a response rate of 29 to 40% and a median overall survival of 6 to 18 months. Unfortunately, many patients develop extrahepatic relapse after chemoembolization and intra-arterial chemotherapy.

In the present patient, CT scans of the chest, abdomen, and pelvis revealed multiple enlarged masses in the liver replacing more then 50% of parenchyma. A CT-guided fine needle aspirate of one of the liver lesions showed metastatic melanoma. The patient received four cycles of intrahepatic chemotherapy with doxorubicin. A restaging CT showed no interval change in diffuse metastatic disease in the liver; however, a soft tissue mass had developed in the anterior lateral chest wall associated with a pathological fracture of the fifth rib. The patient then received hyperfractionated radiation to the chest wall, and his chemotherapy was changed to cisplatin, carmustine, and temozolomide. After two cycles of chemotherapy his LDH had normalized, and a restaging CT scan showed marked improvement of the liver metastases as well as the chest wall mass and adrenal mass. The patient is currently undergoing his fifth cycle of chemotherapy and reports that he is feeling very well. He continues to work full time.

Clinical Pearls

1. Ocular melanomas have a purely hematogenous pattern of dissemination.
2. There is no lymphangitic spread due to absence of lymphatics in the eye. The liver is the most common metastatic site.
3. Patients should be followed with physical exams and liver function tests every 3 to 6 months, as well as with an annual chest X-ray and abdominal ultrasound.
4. Relapses often occur after decades.

REFERENCES

1. Eskelin S, Pyrhonen S, Hahka-Kemppinen M, et al: A prognostic model and staging for metastatic uveal melanoma. Cancer 97:465, 2003.
2. Kivelae T, Suciu S, Hansson J, et al: Bleomycin, vincristine, lomustine and dacarbazine (BOLD) in combination with recombinant interferon alpha-2b for metastatic uveal melanoma. Eur J Cancer 39(8):1115-1120, 2003.
3. Schmittel A, Bechrakis NE, Scheilbenbogen C, et al: Prognostic factors for development of metastatic disease in ocular melanoma: 5-year follow-up of 271 patients (abstract). Proc Am Soc Clin Oncol 22:711a, 2003.
4. Leyvraz S, Spataro V, Bauer J, et al: Treatment of ocular melanoma metastatic to the liver by hepatic arterial chemotherapy. J Clin Oncol 15:2589, 1997.
5. Gragoudas ES, Egan KM, Seddon JM, et al: Survival of patients with metastases from uveal melanoma. Ophthalmology 98:383, 1991.
6. Seddon JM, Gradoudas ES, Egan KM, et al: Relative survival rates after alternative therapies for uveal melanoma. Ophthalmology 97:769, 1990.
7. Gallagher RP, Elwood JM, Tootman J, et al: Risk factors for ocular melanoma: Western Canada Melanoma Study. J Natl Cancer Inst 74:775, 1985.
8. Tucker MA, Shields JA, Hartge P, et al: Sunlight exposure as risk factor for intraocular malignant melanoma. N Engl J Med 313:789, 1985.

PATIENT 67

A 46-year-old woman with abnormal vaginal spotting

A 46-year-old woman with no prior medical history reported several months of menses lasting up to 10 days and spotting between her menses. Her initial workup included a biopsy of a 2-cm cervical mass, which revealed squamous cell carcinoma. Two weeks ago she underwent a radical hysterectomy. The patient has been recovering well, with no complications. She presents to clinic for consideration of further treatment.

Physical Examination: General: no acute distress. Vital signs: temperature 36.6°C, pulse 100, blood pressure 120/80 mmHg. Cardiac: regular rate and rhythm, without murmurs. Chest: clear to auscultation bilaterally. Breasts: no masses, skin changes, or nipple discharge. Abdomen: healing incision scar with no erythema, tenderness, or drainage. Pelvic exam: surgically absent cervix and uterus.

Laboratory Findings: Hemoglobin 10.2 g/dL, WBC 5000/μL, platelets 180,000/μL. Coagulation parameters: normal. Biochemistry profile: normal. Liver function tests: unremarkable. Pathology: 2.5-cm mass replacing full thickness of cervix with parametrial extension; no involvement of uterus or any lymph nodes; surgical margins negative; some areas of vascular invasion.

Questions: What stage cervical cancer does the patient have? What treatment is recommended at this point?

Answers: The patient has early nonbulky stage IB cervical cancer. Following hysterectomy, multimodality treatment with concurrent chemotherapy and radiation is recommended.

Discussion: Cervical cancer is staged according to the International Federation of Gynecology and Obstetrics (FIGO) staging system, last updated in 1994. Staging is based on the initial clinical examination as well as the results of the following procedures and studies: colposcopy, endocervical curettage, hysteroscopy, cystoscopy, proctoscopy, intravenous urography, and radiographic imaging of the lungs and skeleton. The TNM staging system is not widely used (required information for TNM staging is usually not available for patients who do not undergo surgery).

According to the FIGO system, stage IA describes microscopic invasive cervical cancer. In stage IA1 lesions, stromal invasion is less than or equal to 3 mm deep and 7 mm wide; stage IA2 describes deeper and wider lesions up to 5 mm and 7 mm, respectively. Stage IB lesions are grossly visible but confined to the cervix and are subdivided into lesions less than 4 cm (stage IB1) and greater than 4 cm (stage IB2).

Cervical cancer grows locally to involve the vagina and parametrial tissues. If the tumor extends beyond the cervix, but not to the pelvic wall or beyond the upper two-thirds of the vagina, it is classified as stage II disease (IIA, vaginal extension; IIB, parametrial invasion). Tumor involving the lower third of the vagina, but not the pelvic wall, is stage IIIA. Stage IIIB disease extends to the pelvic wall and may cause hydronephrosis or a nonfunctioning kidney. Stage IV disease involves adjacent organs (IVA, mucosal involvement of the bladder or rectum; IVB, distant metastasis). This patient has stage IB1 cervical cancer.

In patients whose disease is confined to the cervix (stage I disease), surgery is generally considered curative. Patients with stage IA1 disease may be treated with a cervical conization with close follow-up, or with simple hysterectomy. The risk of nodal metastases increases with the depth of stromal invasion. Thus, patients with stage IA2 to IIA lesions are treated generally with a radical hysterectomy that includes pelvic lymph node dissection and para-aortic lymph node sampling. If surgery is medically contraindicated, radiation therapy (intracavitary brachytherapy with external-beam radiation to include the pelvic nodes) can also be used for early-stage disease.

Patients with early-stage disease (IA2, IB, IIA) who have positive pelvic lymph nodes, positive margins, or parametrial involvement are considered to be at high risk for recurrent disease and should receive adjuvant therapy. In Southwest Oncology Group (SWOG) trial no. 8797 by Peters and colleagues, such patients were randomized to receive adjuvant radiation versus combined chemotherapy–radiation. Patients receiving chemotherapy concurrently with radiation experienced significantly improved progression-free survival (PFS) and overall survival (OS): projected 4-year PFS was 80% versus 63% for radiation alone; 4-year OS was 81% versus 71% for radiation alone.

Other risk factors for recurrence include tumor invasion of capillary-lymphatic spaces, deep stromal invasion, and large tumor size. Patients with early-stage disease and a combination of these risk factors have been randomized to receive adjuvant radiation therapy after initial surgery. Although the recurrence rate decreased by 44%, there was no clear survival advantage.

This patient with early nonbulky stage IB disease underwent the appropriate initial treatment: radical hysterectomy. The parametrial involvement of her tumor places her at higher risk of recurrence and warrants adjuvant therapy with combined chemotherapy–radiation. Four cycles of cisplatin and fluorouracil are generally administered concurrently with pelvic radiation.

Clinical Pearls

1. Cervical cancer is staged clinically according to the FIGO staging system not the TNM system.

2. Early-stage IA1 through IIA cervical disease can be treated with radical hysterectomy alone.

3. Risk factors associated with higher rates of recurrence include positive surgical margins, parametrial involvement, and/or positive lymph nodes. Such patients should receive adjuvant concurrent chemotherapy–radiation.

REFERENCES

1. Peters WA III, Liu PY, Barrett RJ Jr, et al: Concurrent chemotherapy and pelvic radiation therapy compared with pelvic radiation therapy alone as adjuvant therapy after radical surgery in high-risk early-stage cancer of the cervix. J Clin Oncol 18(8):1606-1613, 2000.
2. Sedlis A, Bundy BN, Rotman MZ, et al: A randomized trial of pelvic radiation therapy versus no further therapy in selected patients with stage 1B carcinoma of the cervix after radical hysterectomy and pelvic lymphadenectomy. Gyn Oncol 73:177-183, 1999.

PATIENT 68

A 45-year-old woman with foul-smelling vaginal
discharge for 2 months

A 45-year-old woman with watery, foul-smelling vaginal discharge of 2-month duration presents to her gynecologist. She also reports occasional vaginal bleeding between menses and after intercourse. She has a history of abnormal Pap smears, most recently 1 year ago, showing atypical squamous cells of unknown significance (ASCUS).

Physical Examination: General: well-appearing, no acute distress. Vital signs: temperature 37°C, pulse 96, blood pressure 106/50 mmHg. Cardiovascular: regular rate and rhythm, without murmurs. Chest: clear to auscultation. Abdomen: no masses, nontender, normal bowel sounds. Pelvic exam under anesthesia: 6-cm cervical lesion with central necrosis, with parametrial extension to the pelvic sidewall.

Laboratory Findings: CBC: hemoglobin 9.8 g/dL, WBC 4000/μL, platelets 120,000/μL; coagulation parameters normal. Biochemistry profile: electrolytes normal. BUN 10, creatinine 0.8. Cervical biopsy: invasive, moderately differentiated squamous cell carcinoma. MRI pelvis: large cervical tumor with bilateral parametrial invasion to sidewall; no lymphadenopathy identified (see Figure).

Questions: What is the clinical stage of the patient's cervical cancer? What is the recommended treatment?

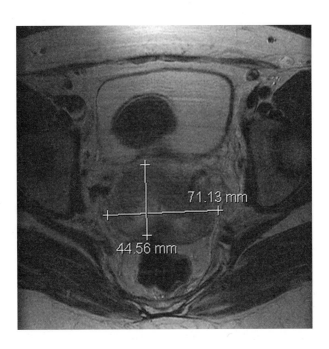

Answers: The patient has stage IIIB cervical cancer. The recommended treatment is concurrent chemotherapy–radiation.

Discussion: In the staging of cervical cancer, locally advanced disease refers to IIB through IVA. Patients with stage IVB have evidence of distant metastasis and are treated with palliative chemotherapy.

In the past, pelvic radiation was the standard therapy for locally advanced disease, with an overall 5-year survival rate of approximately 65%. However, the results of several prospective randomized trials support the use of concurrent chemoradiation with a cisplatin-containing regimen to treat locally advanced disease. In general, a combination of external pelvic and intracavitary radiation totaling 75–85 Gray has been used in these studies. The mechanism of synergy between chemotherapy and radiation is unknown. Chemotherapy may act to inhibit radiation-induced sublethal DNA repair by tumor cells or to promote entry of tumor cells into a radiation-sensitive portion of the cell cycle.

In the Gynecologic Oncology Group (GOG) trial no. 120 reported by Rose and colleagues, patients with stages IIB to IVA were randomized to receive radiation concomitantly with either cisplatin, cisplatin–5-fluorouracil–hydroxyurea, or hydroxyurea alone. All patients received external beam radiation to the pelvis followed by intracavitary brachytherapy. The rate of progression-free survival at 2 years in the cisplatin group was 67%, versus 64% in the group treated with cisplatin–fluorouracil–hydroxyurea, versus 47% in the hydroxyurea group.

In the Radiation Therapy Oncology Group (RTOG) trial no. 9901 by Morris and colleagues, patients with stages IIB to IVA cervical cancer received radiation alone versus radiation and cisplatin–fluorouracil chemotherapy. The median duration of follow-up was 43 months. Overall survival rates were 73% in the group receiving chemoradiation and 58% in the group receiving radiotherapy alone.

Whitney and colleagues conducted a randomized comparison of fluorouracil with cisplatin versus concurrent hydroxyurea–radiotherapy in stages IIB to IVA patients. With a median follow-up of 8.7 years, they reported 43% disease progression in the group receiving cisplatin-based chemotherapy with radiation and 53% disease progression in the group receiving hydroxyurea with radiation.

For the present patient, a reasonable treatment recommendation is definitive radiation (external beam and intracavitary) and weekly cisplatin. The subsequent role of adjuvant hysterectomy after chemoradiation is controversial.

Clinical Pearls

1. Patients with stages IIB to IVA disease should be treated with concurrent chemotherapy–radiation.
2. Definitive radiation includes external beam therapy to the pelvis and/or extended field and intracavitary brachytherapy.
3. Concurrent chemotherapy should be a cisplatin-based regimen.
4. Stage IVB metastatic disease should be treated with palliative chemotherapy.

REFERENCES

1. Keys HM, Bundy BN, Stehman FB, et al: Cisplatin, radiation, and adjuvant hysterectomy compared with radiation and adjuvant hysterectomy for bulky stage IB cervical carcinoma. N Engl J Med 340(15):1154-1161, 1999.
2. Morris M, Eifel PJ, Jiandong L, et al: Pelvic radiation with concurrent chemotherapy compared with pelvic and para-aortic radiation for high-risk cervical cancer. N Engl J Med 340(15):1137-1143, 1999.
3. Rose PG, Bundy BN, Watkins EB: Concurrent cisplatin-based radiotherapy and chemotherapy for locally advanced cervical cancer. N Engl J Med 340(15):1144-1153, 1999.
4. Whitney CW, Sause W, Bundy BN, et al: Randomized comparison of fluorouracil plus cisplatin versus hydroxyurea as an adjunct to radiation therapy in stage IIB-IVA carcinoma of the cervix with negative para-aortic lymph nodes: A Gynecologic Oncology Group and Southwest Oncology Group Study. JCO 17(5):1339-1348, 1999.

PATIENT 69

A 56-year-old woman with hormone-receptor–positive early-stage breast cancer

A 56-year-old postmenopausal woman presents to a medical oncologist after undergoing a mastectomy. She is seeking recommendations regarding adjuvant therapy. A screening mammogram performed 1 month prior revealed a mass in the upper outer quadrant of the left breast. After a core biopsy revealed malignancy, the patient underwent a lumpectomy. Margins were close, so she then underwent left total mastectomy. A sentinel node biopsy was performed at that time. There is no family history of breast cancer. Her past medical history is significant for osteopenia, for which she takes calcium and vitamin D. Review of systems is positive for hot flashes.

Physical Examination: Temperature 36.7°C, pulse 64, blood pressure 122/68 mmHg. General: well nourished. HEENT: no scleral icterus, mucous membranes moist. Neck: no adenopathy. Cardiovascular: regular rate and rhythm, without murmurs. Chest: clear to auscultation, status post left mastectomy with healed scar, right breast without masses. Abdomen: soft, nontender, no organomegaly or masses. Extremities: no axillary adenopathy, no edema or calf tenderness.

Laboratory Findings: Hemoglobin 13 g/dL, WBC 4700/μL, platelets 222,000/μL. Biochemistry profile: normal. Liver function tests: normal. Chest radiograph: normal. Pathology: 4-mm invasive ductal carcinoma, moderately well-differentiated, no lymphovascular invasion, estrogen and progesterone receptors positive, HER2neu not overexpressed, margins negative, sentinel nodes negative by hematoxylin and eosin stain and immunohistochemistry.

Questions: What type of adjuvant therapy is indicated? How will it benefit the patient?

Answers: The patient should consider adjuvant hormonal therapy. Tamoxifen for 5 years is the standard of care for hormone-receptor–positive early-stage tumors and has been proven to decrease the risk of recurrent breast cancer and to improve survival in such patients. Aromatase inhibitors prescribed either instead of or in sequence with tamoxifen are effective as well and can be considered for routine use. The optimal means of incorporating these newer agents (following or replacing tamoxifen) are not yet firmly established.

Discussion: The patient has node-negative, hormone-receptor–positive early-stage breast cancer. The rationale for the administration of systemic adjuvant therapy for patients with early-stage breast cancer is that, despite having undergone surgical removal of all known breast cancer, patients may still harbor microscopic metastases that could, ultimately, develop into clinically evident recurrence and lead to death.

There are two categories of systemic adjuvant therapy: *cytotoxic chemotherapy* and *hormonal therapy*. In 2000, the National Institutes of Health convened a consensus conference to develop guidelines for the administration of adjuvant therapy for early-stage breast cancer. According to these guidelines, adjuvant hormonal therapy should be offered to all patients with hormone-receptor–positive tumors, regardless of age, menopausal status, tumor size, and axillary lymph node status. Cytotoxic chemotherapy is recommended for all women with positive axillary lymph nodes and women with tumors larger than 1 cm.

Based on these guidelines, the patient should consider adjuvant hormonal therapy. The current standard of care for adjuvant hormonal therapy is tamoxifen for 5 years. Tamoxifen is a selective estrogen receptor modulator with antagonistic effects on breast tissue. The recommendation for 5 years of tamoxifen therapy is based largely on the findings of a meta-analysis combining the results of 55 randomized trials of adjuvant tamoxifen therapy. The meta-analysis demonstrates that in hormone receptor–positive patients, 5 years of tamoxifen therapy reduces the risk of breast cancer recurrence by 47% and reduces the risk of death by 26%. These beneficial effects are present regardless of lymph node status, age, and menopausal status, and whether or not cytotoxic chemotherapy is also administered, but the absolute survival benefit is higher for women with higher risk disease, such as those with metastases to ipsilateral lymph nodes. Of note, this meta-analysis demonstrates significantly greater benefit with 5 years of tamoxifen than with shorter courses of therapy. In addition, it demonstrates that the benefits associated with 5 years of tamoxifen therapy persist through 10 years of follow-up, suggesting a carryover effect.

The National Surgical Adjuvant Breast and Bowel Project B-14 trial further investigated the appropriate duration of tamoxifen therapy. This trial compared 5- and 10-year courses of tamoxifen therapy in hormone-receptor–positive, lymph node–negative early-stage breast cancer patients, finding that longer therapy does *not* confer additional benefit. In fact, patients who discontinue tamoxifen after 5 years have improved disease-free survival and a trend toward improved overall survival compared to patients who continue tamoxifen for 10 years, suggesting that 5 years is the most appropriate duration, possibly because tamoxifen resistance, or even dependence, develops over time. Of note, adverse events associated with adjuvant tamoxifen therapy noted in these studies include increased incidence of and death from endometrial cancer, hot flashes, vaginal discharge, irregular menses, thromboembolism, and hospitalization.

Aromatase inhibitors represent new options for adjuvant hormonal therapy for postmenopausal women with early-stage breast cancer. These drugs inhibit the conversion of adrenal androgens to estrogens. Currently available aromatase inhibitors include anastrazole, letrozole, and exemestane. Their efficacy and tolerability in the metastatic breast cancer setting has prompted evaluation of their role in treating hormone receptor–positive early-stage breast cancer in postmenopausal women. Preliminary results of the Arimidex, Tamoxifen, Alone or in Combination (ATAC) trial indicate that 3-year disease-free survival for early-stage breast cancer patients treated with anastrazole is 89.4% in comparison to 87.4% for patients treated with tamoxifen. Four-year results were similar. However, an overall survival advantage for therapy with anastrazole in comparison to tamoxifen has not yet been seen. Furthermore, the optimal duration of adjuvant therapy with anastrazole remains to be determined, and superiority of anastrazole over tamoxifen after adjuvant cytotoxic chemotherapy has not yet been demonstrated. Importantly, the side effects associated with aromatase inhibitors differ from those associated with tamoxifen. The ATAC trial demonstrated that in comparison to tamoxifen, anastrazole is associated with more fractures and musculoskeletal disorders, but with fewer hot flashes, vaginal discharge, stroke, thromboembolism, and endometrial cancer.

In addition to being evaluated as alternatives to tamoxifen for postmenopausal women with hormone-receptor–positive early-stage breast cancer, aromatase inhibitors are being evaluated for use in sequence with tamoxifen. A recent randomized trial demonstrated that treatment with 5 years of letrozole after 5 years of tamoxifen improves 4-year disease-free survival from 87% with tamoxifen alone to 93% with both drugs used in sequence. This study was terminated early (with 5 of 6 planned years of follow-up) based on these findings. Unanswered questions at this time include the optimal duration of letrozole therapy after tamoxifen and the potential long-term toxicities associated with letrozole therapy after tamoxifen. Side effects noted with letrozole in this study were consistent with those noted with anastrazole in the ATAC trial, with musculoskeletal complaints and osteoporosis occurring more frequently in the group receiving letrozole after tamoxifen. In another recent trial assessing the use of aromatase inhibitors in sequence with tamoxifen, postmenopausal women with early-stage estrogen receptor-positive breast cancer treated with 2 to 3 years of tamoxifen were randomized to continuing tamoxifen or switching to exemestane to complete a 5-year course of therapy. After 3 years of follow-up, disease-free survival was 91.5% in the exemestane arm and 86.6% in the tamoxifen arm. Side effects from exemestane in this trial were similar to those observed in the other adjuvant aromatase inhibitor trials described above.

Clearly, research to date indicates that aromatase inhibitors provide an alternative or addition to tamoxifen as adjuvant hormonal therapy for hormone-receptor–positive early-stage breast cancer. However, the many as yet unanswered questions concerning their use make it reasonable to continue to select tamoxifen as initial adjuvant therapy. Physicians are urged to review the available data with their patients and to individualize treatment decisions.

The present patient began a 5-year program of tamoxifen. Thus far, she has not experienced a recurrence of disease.

Clinical Pearls

1. The rationale for the administration of systemic adjuvant therapy for patients with early-stage breast cancer is that, despite having undergone surgical removal of all known breast cancer, patients may still harbor microscopic metastases that could ultimately develop into clinically evident recurrence and lead to death.

2. Adjuvant hormonal therapy should be considered for all women with hormone-receptor–positive early-stage breast cancers.

3. Treatment with tamoxifen for 5 years is currently the standard of care for adjuvant hormonal therapy.

4. Aromatase inhibitors represent newer options for adjuvant hormonal therapy in postmenopausal women and may be used instead of or in sequence with tamoxifen.

REFERENCES

1. Coombes RC, Hall E, Gibson LJ, et al: A randomized trial of exemestane after two to three years of tamoxifen therapy in postmenopausal women with primary breast cancer. N Engl J Med 350(11):1081-1092, 2004.
2. Goss PE, Ingle JN, Martino S, et al: A randomized trial of letrozole in postmenopausal women after five years of tamoxifen therapy for early-stage breast cancer. N Engl J Med 349(19):1793-1802, 2003.
3. Baum M, Budzar AU, Cuzick J, et al: Anastrazole alone or in combination with tamoxifen versus tamoxifen alone for adjuvant treatment of postmenopausal women with early breast cancer: First results of the ATAC randomised trial. Lancet 359(9324):2131-2139, 2002.
4. Winer EP, Hudis C, Burstein HJ, et al: American Society of Clinical Oncology technology assessment on the use of aromatase inhibitors a adjuvant therapy for women with hormone receptor-positive breast cancer: Status report 2002. J Clin Oncol 20(15):3317-3327, 2002.
5. Anonymous: National Institutes of Health Consensus Development Conference Statement: Adjuvant Therapy for Breast Cancer, November 1–3, 2000. J Natl Cancer Inst 93(13):979-989, 2001.
6. Early Breast Cancer Trialists' Collaborative Group: Tamoxifen for early breast cancer: An overview of the randomised trials. Lancet 351(9114):1451-1467, 1998.
7. Fisher B, Dignam J, Bryant J, et al: Five versus more than five years of tamoxifen for breast cancer patients with negative lymph nodes and estrogen receptor–positive tumors. J Natl Cancer Inst 88(21):1529-1542, 1996.

PATIENT 70

A 61-year-old man status post nephrectomy with abdominal pain and anemia

A 61-year-old man with a past medical history significant for transitional cell cancer status post-nephrectomy presented with a right shoulder cyst. The cyst was removed and found to be a sebaceous neoplasm. A left cheek lesion subsequently developed and was also removed. Now, 2 months later, he presents with anemia and right upper quadrant pain. The patient's family history is significant for paternal death from gastric cancer at age 52.

Physical Examination:　Temperature 36.4°C, pulse 64, blood pressure 116/70 mmHg. General: chronically ill-appearing. Cardiovascular: regular rate and rhythm, systolic ejection murmur. Chest: clear to auscultation bilaterally. Abdomen: tender to deep palpation RUQ, bowel sounds decreased. Extremities: no peripheral edema. Skin: multiple cyst-like lesions on upper chest area.

Laboratory Findings:　WBC 8200/μL, hemoglobin 9.1 g/dL, platelets 232,000/μL, creatinine 1.2 mg/dL, BUN 15 mg/dL. Pathology of cheek lesion: atypical sebaceous neoplasm. Abdominal CT scan: mass in the hepatic flexure of his transverse colon.

Course:　After surgical removal of the colonic mass, the patient's skin lesions disappear without further intervention.

Questions:　From which syndrome is the patient suffering? What will the pathology of the colonic mass most likely show?

Answers: The patient is suffering from Muir-Torre syndrome. Pathology will most likely reveal adenocarcinoma of the colon.

Discussion: The Muir-Torre syndrome is a variant of *hereditary nonpolyposis colorectal cancer* (HNPCC) and refers to patients with HNPCC who also develop benign or malignant sebaceous gland tumors. In 1967, Muir and Torre each reported on patients with multiple cutaneous tumors and visceral malignancies. Muir-Torre syndrome is a familial cancer syndrome that combines at least one sebaceous neoplasm (sebaceous adenoma, sebaceous epithelioma, or sebaceous carcinoma) and at least one visceral malignancy (usually gastrointestinal or genitourinary). The syndrome is inherited in an autosomal dominant manner with a high degree of penetrance and variable expression. In many patients the cancers tend to have a nonaggressive course. However, metastatic disease develops in approximately 60% of patients, with a 50% 10-year survival. The syndrome occurs in both sexes, with a male-to-female ratio of 3:2. The median age is 53 years, but there is a wide age variation.

The most common visceral neoplasm in Muir-Torre syndrome is colorectal cancer, occurring in almost one-half of patients. The tumors are usually proximal to the splenic flexure. The second most common site is the genitourinary tract. A wide variety of other cancers, including breast cancer, lymphoma, and chondrosarcoma, are reported.

Another variant of HNPCC is *Turcot's syndrome*, which is associated with glioblastoma multiforme. HNPCC is more common than familial adenomatous polyposis, accounting for about 1 to 5% of all colorectal adenocarcinomas. It is characterized by early-onset colorectal cancer, multiple colorectal cancers, and colorectal cancers that are mostly located in the proximal colon. Associated are adenocarcinomas of the ovary, pancreas, breast, bile duct, endometrium, stomach, genitourinary tract, and small bowel.

HNPCC can be divided into *Lynch I and Lynch II syndromes*. Lynch I syndrome, or hereditary site-specific colon cancer, occurs at an early age, usually in the proximal colon. Lynch II syndrome, or cancer family syndrome, is associated not only with colon cancer but also ovary, stomach, small bowel, hepatobiliary system, and renal pelvis or ureter cancer. The most common is endometrial carcinoma, which develops in up to 43% of females in affected families. However, the distinction between Lynch I and Lynch II is becoming less clear as more families are studied.

Tumors arising in patients with HNPCC appear to evolve from colorectal adenomas, which can appear flat rather then polypoid. The polyps tend to have villous histology, which is associated with an increased risk of malignant transformation compared to tubular histology. Tumors in patients with HNPCC are generally poorly differentiated. However, the overall 5-year survival rate in affected patients is better than that seen in sporadic colorectal cancer, suggesting a different biology. The mean age at initial HNPCC diagnosis is 48 years, with some patients presenting in their twenties. Nearly 70% of first lesions arise proximal to the splenic flexure, and approximately 10% will have synchronous or metachronous cancers.

Germ-line mutations in one of six DNA mismatch repair genes appear to be the underlying genetic defect in most kindreds with HNPCC. Commercial testing is available for the mismatch repair gene abnormalities hMSH2 and hMLH1. The available assays have sensitivities greater than 95%. Individuals with germ-line mutations on one of the HNPCC genes are at high risk (70-90%) for developing colorectal cancer. The risk appears to be higher in men than in woman (80-90% vs 30%). Woman who are HNPCC gene carriers also have a high risk of developing endometrial cancer (39%) and ovarian cancer (9%).

The term *microsatellite instability* refers to the expansion or contraction of short repeated DNA sequences that are caused by insertion or deletion of repeated units. The phenomenon of microsatellite instability is present in 90% of tumors from patients with HNPCC and in only 12% of sporadic colon cancer cases. The presence of microsatellite instability in tumor tissue suggests that a defect in a DNA mismatch repair gene may be present. Patients whose tumors demonstrate microsatellite instability have improved survival but decreased responsiveness to chemotherapy.

The present patient was found to have locally advanced adenocarcinoma of the colon with lymph node involvement and is currently recovering adjuvant 5-FU–based chemotherapy. He is tolerating his chemotherapy very well.

Clinical Pearls

1. Hereditary nonpolyposis colorectal cancer (HNPCC) is more likely to be a signet-ring type, and it is poorly differentiated with extensive inflammation.

2. HNPCC tumors are usually located in the proximal colon.

3. The survival for colorectal cancer patients with HNPCC is better on a stage-for-stage basis than for patients with sporadic cases.

4. Patients whose tumors demonstrate microsatellite instability may have improved survival but decreased responsiveness to chemotherapy.

REFERENCES

1. Gryfe R, Kim H, Hsieh ETK, et al: Tumor microsatellite instability and clinical outcome in young patients with colorectal cancer. N Engl J Med 342:69, 2000.

2. Ribic CM, Sargent DJ, Moore MJ, et al: Tumor microsatellite-instability status as a predictor of benefit from fluorouracil-based adjuvant chemotherapy for colon cancer. N Engl J Med 349:3, 2000.

3. Aaltonen LA, Salovaara R, Kristo P, et al: Incidence of hereditary nonpolyposis colorectal cancer and the feasibility of molecular screening for this disease. N Engl J Med 338:1481, 1998.

4. Burt RW, DiSario JA, Cannon-Albright L: Genetics of colon cancer: Impact of inheritance on colon cancer risk. Annu Rev Med 46:371, 1995.

5. International Multicentre Pooled Analysis of Colon Cancer Trials (IMPACT) Investigators. Efficacy of adjuvant fluorouracil and folinic acid in colon cancer. Lancet 345:939-944, 1995.

6. Watson P, Lynch HT: Extracolonic cancer in hereditary nonpolyposis colorectal cancer. Cancer 71:677, 1993.

7. Mecklin JP, Jarvinen HJ: Tumor spectrum in cancer family syndrome (hereditary nonpolyposis colorectal cancer). Cancer 68:1109, 1991.

PATIENT 71

A 24-year-old woman with multiple metastases following stillbirth

A 24-year-old woman experiences a stillbirth at 27 weeks' gestation. One week later symptoms of thyroid storm develop, and she is started on propylthiouracil (PTU) and propranolol. After several days pass, she presents with nausea and visual disturbances. She is passing tissue from her vagina.

Physical Examination: General: fatigued-appearing, no acute distress. Temperature 36.6°C, pulse 96, blood pressure 145/70 mmHg. HEENT: oropharynx clear, sclerae anicteric. Lymph nodes: no cervical, supraclavicular, axillary, or inguinal lymphadenopathy. Cardiovascular: regular rate and rhythm, no murmurs. Chest: clear throughout. Abdomen: soft, mildly tender throughout, without rebound or peritoneal signs.

Laboratory Findings: Complete blood count and extended chemistries: normal. β-hCG level: 8,894,060. CT scan: masses in lungs and liver; bilateral theca lutein cysts; enlarged uterus and pelvic soft tissue mass (see Figure). Brain MRI: scattered small lesions in occipital lobe. Pathology from placenta: abnormal.

Questions: What is the most likely diagnosis? What is the recommended course of treatment?

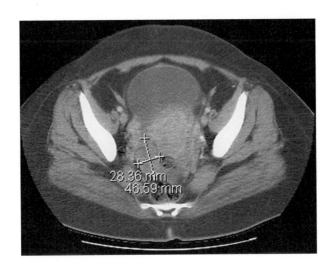

Answers: Choriocarcinoma is the most likely diagnosis. The patient needs immediate hospitalization and treatment with systemic chemotherapy.

Discussion: Gestational trophoblastic disease (GTD) refers to a group of rare tumors (1–2 per 1000 pregnancies worldwide) that arise as a result of abnormal conception. All are characterized by elevated β-human chorionic gonadotropin (β-hCG) levels, and they are remarkable in that most are exquisitely sensitive to chemotherapy: cure rates of 90% can be achieved even in the setting of metastatic disease. Tumors included in this heading include hydatidiform moles (complete or partial, also known as molar pregnancies), invasive moles, choriocarcinomas, and placental site trophoblastic tumors (PSTT).

Hydatidiform moles arise after conception and represent the abnormal development of chorionic villi within the placental tissue. Hydatidiform moles are classified as either complete or partial, based on morphology, karyotype, and pathology. No identifiable embryonic tissue is evident in a complete mole. Embryonic tissue may be present in a partial mole, but any fetal formation is characterized by growth retardation and multiple genetic abnormalities. An invasive mole is a hydatidiform mole that has invaded the myometrium. These often present as persistent disease after treatment of a hydatidiform mole.

Gestational choriocarcinomas can present dramatically, as illustrated by this case. They can arise after any gestational event (spontaneous abortion, molar pregnancy, ectopic pregnancy, term pregnancy) and develop from any type of trophoblastic tissue. PSTTs arise from the implantation site of intermediate trophoblasts after a full-term pregnancy or nonmolar pregnancy. They are unusual in that they can arise up to several years after an antecedent pregnancy, produce lower levels of β-hCG, and are less sensitive to chemotherapy.

The diagnosis of a GTD is made usually in a woman with vaginal bleeding who believes she might be pregnant or who was recently pregnant. Very high serum β-hCG levels are typical of this disease. A positive serum β-hCG must always be confirmed by a urine pregnancy test before initiating any therapy, because heterophile antibodies can cause false-positive serum levels. Patients with hydatidiform moles may also exhibit uterine size larger than gestational age, hyperemesis, hyperthyroidism (secondary to stimulation of the thyroid hormone (TSH) receptor by β-hCG or other placental proteins), theca lutein cysts, and early preeclampsia (< 20 weeks). Choriocarcinomas are clinically aggressive and may present with vaginal hemorrhage, respiratory distress due to tumor emboli or metastatic disease, and, rarely, intracerebral hemorrhage due to metastases from this vascular tumor.

When GTD is suspected clinically, an ultrasound evaluation is often enough to confirm a suspected diagnosis of a hydatidiform mole. The distinction between a mole and choriocarcinoma can be suspected based on clinical presentation. The final diagnosis is confirmed upon pathology after a dilation and curettage (D&C). Once the diagnosis of GTD has been made, further staging should be performed using a CT scan of the chest, abdomen, and pelvis. An MRI of the brain is indicated in patients with hydatidiform moles, if there is evidence of lung or vaginal metastases, and in all cases of choriocarcinoma.

Treatment depends on the type of GTD and prognostic factors. Patients with complete or partial hydatidiform moles can be offered either a D&C, if they wish to preserve fertility, or a hysterectomy, if they plan no future child-bearing. Of note, if a patient is Rh-negative, she should be given RhoGAM when she undergoes D&C to prevent alloimmunization. Close monitoring of β-hCG levels after either procedure is crucial. Levels should be drawn weekly until they are undetectable for 3 weeks, then monthly for 6 months, then yearly for 1 to 3 years. If there is a plateau or rise in the β-hCG levels, this is indicative of either an invasive mole (75%) or choriocarcinoma (25%). At this point, patients undergo staging and evaluation of prognostic factors using the modified WHO scoring system (see Table). Patients with scores greater than or equal to 8 are considered to have high-risk disease. Low- and intermediate-risk invasive moles (scores ≤8) can be treated with single-agent methotrexate, a regimen that is well tolerated and has a good long-term safety profile. The use of methotrexate as a first-line drug is favored over single-agent dactinomycin, because alopecia may occur with the latter. Evaluation and treatment of high-risk disease and all choriocarcinomas must be initiated urgently and often requires immediate hospitalization for systemic therapy with EMA/CO (etoposide, methotrexate, and dactinomycin in week 1; cyclophosphamide and vincristine in week 2).

World Health Organization Prognostic Index Score for Gestational Trophoblastic Disease

Prognostic Factors	Score[a]			
	0	1	2	4
Age	≤ 35	> 35	—	—
Antecedent pregnancy	Hydatidiform mole	Abortion	Term	—
Interval[b]	< 4	4–6	7–12	> 12
hCG	< 10^3	10^3–10^4	10^4–10^5	> 10^5
Largest tumor, including uterine tumor	—	3–5 cm	> 5 cm	—
Site of metastases	—	Spleen, kidney	GI tract	Brain, liver
Number of metastases identified	—	1–4	4–8	> 8
Prior chemotherapy	—	—	Single drug	Two or more

[a]The total score for a patient is obtained by adding the individual scores for each prognostic factor. Total score 0–8 = low risk; greater than 8 = high risk.

[b]Time interval (months) between end of antecedent pregnancy and start of chemotherapy.

hCG = human chorionic gonadotrophin; GI = gastrointestinal.

Approximately 15% of patients who have a clinical presentation similar to the present patient will die early during the course of their treatment, usually from pulmonary hemorrhage. Some clinicians, therefore, advocate that a "slow" approach should be taken when first initiating therapy, with the intention of not lysing the disease too quickly.

All patients receiving systemic therapy should continue to be treated for three to four cycles (6–8 weeks) after normalization of β-hCG levels, regardless of diagnosis or risk. Beta-hCG levels must be checked weekly during therapy. A plateau or rise in levels is considered to be a treatment failure. Patients with an invasive mole who are resistant to methotrexate, but are still considered low risk and have a β-hCG less than 100, can be salvaged with single-agent dactinomycin. Otherwise, they need additional therapy with EMA/CO. Patients who are resistant to EMA/CO can be salvaged with EMA/EP (etoposide, methotrexate, and dactinomycin in week 1; etoposide and cisplatin in week 2). PSTTs have a higher risk of recurrence and are more resistant to chemotherapy. All patients with PSTT should undergo a hysterectomy, after which early introduction of a platinum regimen, such as EMA/EP, can be used.

Fertility is an issue that often arises in patients being treated for this disease. It is recommended to delay trying to become pregnant for 1 to 2 years after treatment of GTD. This encompasses the time frame during which patients are at the highest risk for disease recurrence (and during which there should be close surveillance, including monitoring of β-hCG levels). The use of either oral contraceptives or barrier methods is recommended during this period of close observation. The discussed combination chemotherapy regimens used in this disease do not carry a high risk of infertility, although they may accelerate the onset of menopause.

The present patient experienced a complicated course of therapy. She was immediately admitted to a hospital and received a dose of EMA with high doses of methotrexate administered due to her central nervous system (CNS) involvement. She experienced a major response with a decline in her β-hCG levels to 116,066 after one cycle of EMA. Due to significant thrombocytopenia, pulmonary edema, and the concern for pulmonary hemorrhage, her first week of CO was held. The patient, ultimately, received four cycles of EMA/CO, after which her β-hCG levels reached a plateau. She was therefore switched to EMA/EP with a further decline in levels but complicated by acute renal failure, severe mucositis, and prolonged neutropenia requiring hospitalization. Her β-hCG levels remained mildly elevated, and she therefore received consolidation with three cycles of carboplatin and paclitaxel, after which her β-hCG levels became undetectable. She has now completely recovered from her treatment and has been disease-free on oral contraceptives for 2 years.

Clinical Pearls

1. Choriocarcinoma is a medical emergency requiring immediate evaluation and treatment.

2. Elevated serum β-hCG levels must be confirmed with a urine hCG test prior to initiating therapy for gestational trophoblastic disease.

3. β-hCG levels must be closely monitored during therapy to document response. Observation of β-hCG levels is recommended for 1 to 2 years following treatment.

REFERENCES

1. Altieri A, Franceschi S, Ferlay J, et al: Epidemiology and aetiology of gestational trophoblastic diseases. Lancet 4:670-678, 2003.
2. Bentley RC: Pathology of gestational trophoblastic disease. Clin Obstet Gynecol 46:513-522, 2003.
3. Wright JD, Mutch DG: Treatment of high-risk gestational trophoblastic tumors. Clin Obstet Gynecol 46:593-606, 2003.
4. McNeish IA, Stickland S, Holden L, et al: Low-risk persistent gestational trophoblastic disease: Outcome after initial treatment with low-dose methotrexate and folinic acid from 1992 to 2000. J Clin Oncol 20:1838-1844, 2002.
5. Cohn D, Herzog TJ: Gestational trophoblastic diseases: New standards for therapy. Curr Opin Oncol 12:492-496, 2000.

PATIENT 72

A 58-year-old man with a left thigh mass

A 58-year-old man was in his usual state of health until he noted a burning sensation and swelling at the posterior aspect of his left thigh. He denies any trauma. Initially, he did not experience any focal weakness, pain, or numbness. However, over several weeks his symptoms progressed, with pain radiating down his leg, exacerbated by walking.

Physical Examination: General: well-nourished, no acute distress. Vital signs: temperature 37°C, blood pressure 124/82 mmHg, pulse 96. Cardiovascular: regular rate and rhythm, without murmurs. Chest: clear to auscultation bilaterally. Extremities: left posterior thigh notable for palpable firm mass, 16 cm × 12 cm, with associated erythema; negative Homans' sign.

Laboratory Findings: Liver function tests: normal. Core biopsy immunohistochemistry: diffusely positive vimentin, focally positive smooth-muscle actin (SMA), negative desmin, negative S100 protein, negative cytokeratin.

Questions: What is the most likely diagnosis? What additional diagnostic studies should be performed prior to recommending treatment?

Answers: The patient has a high-grade soft-tissue sarcoma. Recommended diagnostic studies include an MRI of the thigh to assess the extent of local disease and a chest CT scan to rule out metastatic involvement.

Discussion: The presentation of this patient is typical of high-grade soft-tissue sarcoma (STS): a painless, growing soft tissue mass of a lower extremity, arising in a patient over age 50. In adults, STS is more common than sarcomas of bone (the opposite is true in children). Most forms of STS arise spontaneously within an extremity, usually a lower rather than an upper extremity. STS is also seen (in decreasing order of frequency) within the abdominal cavity/ retroperitoneum, trunk/thoracic region, and head/neck.

The initial diagnostic imaging of choice is MRI to differentiate a soft-tissue tumor from adjacent structures. There are more than 50 different sub-types of STS, and pathological interpretation is useful in determining appropriate therapy. A core biopsy of STS will be consistent with connective tissue immunohistochemistry, for example, with positive vimentin and SMA. Approximately 15% of sarcomas are associated with specific chromosomal translocations, including Ewing's sarcoma/primitive neuroendocrine tumor t(11;22), clear-cell sarcoma t(12;22), and desmoplastic small-round cell tumor t(11;22). Prognostic features include sarcoma grade and histological subtype. There are multiple systems for assessing sarcoma grade, including scales ranging from low- to intermediate- to high-grade soft-tissue sarcoma and grading scales from 1 to 4. The American Joint Committee on Cancer's soft-tissue sarcoma staging takes into account the size of the primary tumor (> 5 cm) and location/extent of invasion (of investing fascia).

Surgery is the principal treatment for localized STS. Limb or function-sparing surgery combined with radiation has been shown to be as good as amputation alone, and thus the former is preferred to preserve function. Radiation therapy for STS to the primary tumor site is the standard of care for all extremity or truncal sarcomas greater than 5 cm, independent of grade. The role of adjuvant chemotherapy for localized STS remains controversial.

The most common site of metastasis is the lungs. Therefore, chest CT is warranted when primary lesions are felt to have metastatic potential (i.e., > 5 cm). The treatment of metastatic STS is palliative (not curative) and may involve systemic chemotherapy (typically with anthracyclines and ifosfamide).

The present patient proceeded to surgery for successful resection of his tumor, and his lower extremity function remained intact. Following his postoperative recovery, he underwent radiation therapy to the thigh.

Clinical Pearls

1. Most soft-tissue sarcomas (STS) in adults arise in the extremities. The most common site of metastasis is the lungs.

2. Approximately 15% of the time, soft-tissue sarcomas are associated with specific chromosomal translocations (more than any other type of solid tumor).

3. Surgery is the principal treatment for soft-tissue sarcomas in adults. Limb or function-sparing surgery combined with radiation is usually preferred over amputation to preserve function.

4. Metastatic STS is treated with palliative chemotherapy, typically with anthracyclines and ifosfamide.

REFERENCES
1. Bennicelli JL, Barr FG: Chromosomal translocations and sarcomas. Curr Opin Oncol 14:412-419, 2002.
2. Brennan MF, Alektiar K, Maki RG: Soft tissue sarcoma. In DeVita VT Jr, Hellman S, Rosenberg S (eds): Cancer: Principles and Practice of Oncology, 6th ed. Philadelphia, Lippincott, Williams & Wilkins, 2001, pp 1841-1891.
3. Singer S, Demetri, Baldini E: Management of soft-tissue sarcomas: An overview and update. Lancet 1:75-85, 2000.
4. Sarcoma Meta-Analysis Collaboration: Adjuvant chemotherapy for adult soft tissue sarcoma of adults: Meta-analysis of individual data. Lancet 350:1647-1654, 1997.

PATIENT 73

An 81-year-old woman with weight loss and a gastric mass

An 81-year-old woman presents to her physician with a 9-month history of progressive weight loss and early satiety. Her past medical history is significant for psoriatic arthropathy and moderate to severe kyphosis.

Physical Examination: Temperature 36.6°C, pulse 80, blood pressure 130/70 mmHg. Lymph nodes: no peripheral adenopathy. Abdomen: no hepatosplenomegaly or masses palpable. Musculoskeletal: severe kyphosis.

Laboratory Findings: CBC: normal. Biochemistry profile: normal. CT scan of abdomen: 6 cm, smoothly ovulated mass involving posterior body of stomach (see Figure). Endoscopy and biopsy of mass: dense atypical lymphoid infiltrate, staining positively for CD20; CD5, CD10; cyclin D1 stains negative.

Questions: What is the most likely diagnosis? What additional stains may predict response to initial therapy?

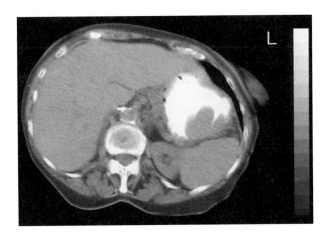

Answers: Gastric mucosa-associated lymphoid tissue (MALT) lymphoma is the most likely diagnosis. A special stain for *Helicobacter pylori* is required.

Discussion: Although the stomach is the most common site for extra nodal marginal zone B-cell lymphoma, other sites, such as salivary gland, thyroid, and lung, may also be involved. Chronic inflammations or infections at these sites include *H. pylori* in the stomach, follicular bronchiectasis in the lung, Sjögren's disease in the salivary gland, and Hashimoto's thyroiditis. Chronic stimulation of T-cells at these sites is thought to result in cytokine release, stimulating B-cells in the marginal zone and leading to the production of a clonal B-cell population. In gastric MALT, there is a 92% association with *H. pylori* infection.

The clinical symptoms at presentation include epigastric pain, dyspepsia, anorexia, nausea, and gastrointestinal bleeding. Staging procedures should include a CT scan of the chest, abdomen, and pelvis; upper GI endoscopy with multiple biopsies; and special stains for *H. pylori*. At the molecular level, up to 40% of gastric MALT lymphomas have the t(11;18) translocation. This translocation is associated with BCL-10 overexpression and is seen more commonly in tumors disseminated beyond the stomach.

The initial treatment for gastric MALT should consist of antibiotic therapy to eradicate *H. pylori*. An example of such an antibiotic regimen is clarithromycin, metronidazole, and omeprazole twice daily for 14 days. Antibiotic therapy causes remission in 60 to 80% of patients treated. Initial failure to eradicate *H. pylori* should prompt a second course of treatment with a different antibiotic regimen. However, tumors with the t(11;18) translocation are usually no longer "antigen driven" by *H. pylori*. This translocation strongly predicts failure to respond to antibiotics, as does disease that has spread to regional lymph nodes.

Patients who fail to respond to two courses of antibiotics should have repeat biopsies to exclude the possibility of transformation to a large-cell lymphoma. Treatment options for nonresponding patients include local treatment, such as gastrectomy or gastric irradiation. Single-agent chemotherapy with chlorambucil or cyclophosphamide is effective, but recent encouraging results with the use of single-agent rituximab has led to this agent being used more commonly than traditional chemotherapy. For transformed disease, combination chemotherapy with rituximab, cyclophosphamide, doxorubicin vincristine, and prednisone (R-CHOP) would be a standard approach.

In the present patient, staining for *H. pylori* was negative. Her gastric lymphoma failed to respond to two courses of antibiotics; therefore, referral to radiation oncology was requested. However, her left kidney was in close proximity to her stomach due to severe kyphosis, and she was not offered gastric irradiation. She is currently receiving single-agent rituximab with a good response.

Clinical Pearls

1. In gastric MALT, the association with *H. pylori* infection is greater than 90%.
2. Up to 40% of gastric MALT lymphomas have the t(11;18) translocation. This translocation strongly predicts failure to respond to antibiotics.
3. Antibiotic therapy causes remission in 60 to 80% of patients treated.
4. Treatment options for patients who fail to respond to two courses of antibiotics include local treatment, such as gastric irradiation.

REFERENCE

Schechter NR, Yahalom J: Low-grade MALT lymphoma of the stomach: A review of treatment options. Int J Radiat Oncol Biol Phys 46(5):1093-1103, 2000.

PATIENT 74

A 35-year-old woman with bright red blood per rectum

A 35-year-old woman with no significant medical history has experienced intermittent bright red blood per rectum for several weeks. Pain with defecation has worsened progressively during this time. In the last week prior to her clinical presentation, she developed the sensation of a mass in the anal area. The patient has no history of sexually transmitted diseases or anogenital warts.

Physical Examination: Temperature 37°C, blood pressure 98/65 mmHg, pulse 92. General: well-developed; no acute distress. HEENT: anicteric, oropharynx clear, no adenopathy. Chest: clear to auscultation bilaterally. Abdomen: normal active bowel sounds, soft, nontender, nondistended, no organomegaly. Rectal: nodular mass palpable on anterior anal canal about 1 to 2 cm from anal margin. Extremities: no clubbing, cyanosis, or edema.

Laboratory Findings: Unremarkable CBC, biochemistry profile, hepatic function panel, and coagulation panel. Endorectal ultrasound: 2-cm nodular ulcerated mass just distal to anorectal ring. Biopsy of anal mass: squamous cell carcinoma, poorly differentiated.

Questions: What are the risk factors for anal cancer? What is the correct initial therapy for the patient?

Answers: Anogenital warts and human papillomavirus (especially type 16) are strong risk factors. Other risk factors include prior sexually transmitted disease, receptive anal intercourse, chronic immunosuppression after solid organ transplantation, and probably smoking. Hemorrhoids and anal fissures do *not* increase the risk of anal cancer. Neoadjuvant chemoradiation is the best initial therapy for the patient.

Discussion: There are about 4000 cases per year of anal cancer in the United States. Eighty percent to 85% are squamous cell carcinomas. About 15% of anal canal tumors are adenocarcinomas, which are treated as rectal cancer. Rare histologies include melanoma, neuroendocrine carcinoma, and sarcoma.

Anal *canal* carcinomas must be distinguished from anal *margin* tumors, which are considered skin cancers and treated with local excision. For larger tumors of the anal canal, the standard of care for many years was abdominoperineal resection (APR) with permanent colostomy, yielding 5-year overall survival rates of 40 to 70%. The current standard of care is to reserve APR for patients in whom chemoradiation fails to control the disease. Two randomized clinical trials have compared chemoradiation versus radiation alone as initial therapy for this disease. Both trials found that *neoadjuvant chemoradiation* spares many patients from colostomy and does not compromise overall survival.

Bartelink and colleagues randomized 110 patients with T_3/T_4 tumors or positive lymph nodes to either chemoradiation or radiation alone. The chemotherapy regimen was 5-fluorouracil plus mitomycin. 45cGy radiation was administered over 5 weeks followed by a boost. After median follow-up of 3.5 years, the local control rate was 58% in the chemotherapy plus radiation group and 39% in the radiation therapy only group.

A larger British study yielded similar results: 585 patients were randomized to radiation therapy alone or radiation therapy with concurrent 5-fluorouracil and mitomycin. Median follow-up was 3.5 years. Relative risk of colostomy was 0.56 in the combined arm compared with radiation alone. There was no significant difference in overall survival between the two treatment arms in either of these trials. Both trials support the principle that chemoradiation spares a significant portion of patients from undergoing APR with colostomy and does not compromise overall survival.

Flam and colleagues reported that colostomy-free survival rates drop significantly if the mitomycin is omitted from the chemoradiotherapy. Therefore, chemoradiation with *5-fluorouracil plus mitomycin* remains the standard of care. Mitomycin is associated with significant toxicity and is not thought to be a radiosensitizing drug. Cisplatin is known to be an effective radiosensitizing agent. Current randomized clinical trials will help determine whether the combination of 5-fluorouracil plus cisplatin is superior to 5-fluorouracil plus mitomycin as neoadjuvant chemoradiation for anal canal cancer. Radiation could be administered in 28 fractions of 180 cGy/day, for total dose 4500–5040 cGy. Radiation ports should include inguinal lymph nodes. Chemotherapy would be mitomycin (8–10 mg/m^2 on day 1 of weeks 1 and 5) and 5-fluorouracil (1000 mg/m^2 daily for 4 or 5 days on weeks 1 and 5).

The present patient received concurrent chemoradiation with 5-fluoruracil and mitomycin. She experienced local recurrence and underwent surgical resection.

Clinical Pearls

1. Adenocarcinoma of the anal canal is treated like rectal cancer.

2. Anal margin tumors are considered to be skin tumors and are treated with local excision.

3. For anal canal squamous cell carcinoma, chemoradiation with 5-fluorouracil and mitomycin spares a significant fraction of patients from abdominoperineal resection with colostomy and does not compromise survival.

REFERENCES

1. Esiashvili N, Landry J, Matthew RH: Carcinoma of the anus: Strategies in management. Oncologist 7:188-199, 2002.
2. Ryan DP, Compton CC, Mayer RJ: Carcinoma of the anal canal. N Engl J Med 342:792-800, 2000.
3. Bartelink H, Roelofsen F, Eschwege F, et al: Concomitant radiotherapy and chemotherapy is superior to radiotherapy alone in the treatment of locally advanced anal cancer: Results of a phase III randomized trial of the European Organization for Research and Treatment of Cancer Radiotherapy and Gastrointestinal Cooperative Groups. J Clin Oncol 15:2040-2049, 1997.
4. Flam M, John M, Pajak TF, et al: Role of mitomycin in combination with fluorouracil and radiotherapy, and of salvage chemoradiation in the definitive nonsurgical treatment of epidermoid carcinoma of the anal canal: Results of a phase III randomized intergroup study. J Clin Oncol 14:2527-2539, 1996.
5. UKCCCR Anal Cancer Working Party: Epidermoid anal cancer: Results from the UKCCCR randomized trial of radiotherapy alone versus radiotherapy, 5-fluorouracil, and mitomycin. Lancet 348:1049-1054, 1996.

PATIENT 75

A 74-year-old man with hepatitis B and hepatocellular carcinoma with recurrent disease status post partial hepatectomy

A 74-year-old Russian man with a history of hepatitis B was found to have hepatocellular carcinoma (HCC) during routine screening. He underwent partial hepatectomy for local disease but experienced intrahepatic recurrence 2 years later. Despite local therapy, including ethanol injection and hepatic artery embolization, metastatic disease to the parietal bone developed during the following year. This isolated metastasis was resected, but within 12 months he experienced increasing abdominal pain and was found to have recurrent disease within segment 1 of the liver.

Physical Examination: Temperature 37.4°C, blood pressure 135/75 mmHg, pulse 84. General: well-nourished. HEENT: mild scleral icterus, posterior scalp scar well healed, no adenopathy. Cardiovascular: regular rate and rhythm, without murmurs. Chest: clear to auscultation. Abdomen: hepatectomy scar well healed, liver edge palpable 2 cm below the costal margin, no ascites. Extremities: no clubbing, cyanosis, or edema. Skin: no jaundice, spider angiomata, petechiae, or caput medusa.

Laboratory Findings: CBC: normal, platelets 144,000/μL. Biochemistry profile: normal. alpha-fetoprotein: 4000 ng/mL. Total bilirubin: 2.1 mg/dL. Albumin: 3.8 g/dL. PT: 15.1. CT scan of chest, abdomen, and pelvis (see Figure): status post right hepatectomy with hypertrophy of left lobe of liver; two nonenhancing low-attenuation masses within segment 4, smaller than prior studies consistent with prior embolization; stable 2.9 cm × 1.6 cm soft tissue mass adjacent to right lateral resection margin; new hypervascular 2.8 cm × 1.9 cm mass in segment 1, worrisome for new focus of hepatocellular carcinoma.

Questions: What is the significance of viral hepatitis as it pertains to hepatocellular carcinoma? What is the role of chemotherapy for the treatment of hepatocellular carcinoma?

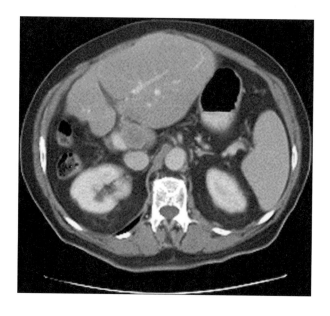

Answers: Viral hepatitis is a major cause of HCC worldwide. Chemotherapy alone is ineffective in the treatment of HCC; however, combination regimens are meeting with some success.

Discussion: Hepatocellular carcinoma is one of the most common malignancies in the world, accounting for one million deaths annually. The highest incidence rates can be found in Western Africa and China, although in the United States the incidence and mortality associated with HCC has nearly doubled between 1981 and 1995. Several risk factors have been identified for the development of HCC; these include viral infections (hepatitis B and C), toxins (e.g., aflatoxin, alcohol-induced cirrhosis), and metabolic disorders (e.g., hemochromatosis, α-1-antitrypsin deficiency, Wilson's disease).

The prevalence of hepatitis B and hepatitis C infection appears to be the most significant cause of HCC worldwide. Hepatitis B incidence shares a geographical distribution with HCC rates. In endemic regions, nearly 90% of HCC patients are infected with hepatitis B virus. The risk of developing HCC increases ninefold in patients with continuing antigenemia and in those with chronic active hepatitis. In addition, the consumption of alcohol in the setting of hepatitis B infection greatly increases the risk of HCC (odds ratio 7.3).

Chronic hepatitis C virus (HCV) infection has emerged as the greatest risk factor for the development of HCC in many parts of the world. In the United States, 3.9 million people are infected with HCV. Eighty-five percent of these patients will develop chronic hepatitis, and 20% of these patients will develop cirrhosis within 10 years of exposure. In contrast to hepatitis B virus (HBV) infection, HCC in patients with HCV occurs almost exclusively in those patients with cirrhosis. Patients with compensated cirrhosis have a 3 to 4% annual incidence of HCC.

Aside from the significance of viral hepatitis in the pathogenesis of HCC, the oncologist is faced with the consequences of chronic liver disease and cirrhosis when contemplating the potential to treat. Therapeutic options are dictated by the extent of disease and the patient's functional hepatic reserve. The TNM staging classification allows for a measure of extent of disease; however, it is limited by the absence of liver function assessment. There are several prognostic scoring systems for HCC that attempt to stratify the severity of cirrhosis, including: the modified Child-Pugh classification, the Okuda system, the Cancer of the Liver Italian Program (CLIP) score, the Barcelona staging classification, and the French prognostic classification. All schemata demonstrate that as hepatic functional reserve declines, so, too, do median and overall survival.

Surgery is the only potential curative therapy in the management of HCC. However, no more than 30% of patients with HCC present with resectable disease. Extrahepatic disease, poor hepatic functional reserve, multifocal disease within the liver, and involvement of the main portal vein are contraindications to resection. Overall 5-year survival rates following partial hepatectomy range from 35 to 50% and should be considered for patients with Child-Pugh class A–B.

Orthotopic liver *transplantation* is associated with an improved survival outcome (5-year survival 70%) in selected patients with small tumors (< 5 cm or fewer than three tumors all < 3 cm) and moderate to severe cirrhosis. However, limited donor availability, significant surgical morbidity, and effects of systemic immunosuppression are concerns for this treatment modality. Interestingly, patients undergoing liver resection with tumors that fit criteria for transplantation had similar survival outcomes to those patients who underwent transplantation.

Several *ablative approaches* exist for the treatment of localized HCC, although there are no randomized controlled trials comparing these to surgery. Local ablative therapies include percutaneous ethanol injection, cryosurgery, radiofrequency ablation, microwave coagulation therapy, and laser coagulation. Intralesional chemotherapy and intratumoral yttrium-90 microsphere injection have been attempted as well. Unfortunately, there are limited data comparing these approaches to one another or to surgery for the treatment of HCC.

High relapse rates after curative therapy for HCC prompted investigation into adjuvant or neoadjuvant systemic therapy. Unfortunately, systemic *chemotherapy* has not demonstrated an improvement in survival in numerous randomized trials when used as primary treatment or in the adjuvant setting. Systemic chemotherapy has been studied in advanced HCC with disappointing results. Agents described with partial response rates approximating 10% include doxorubicin, fluorouracil, and cisplatin. The explanation for the ineffectiveness of chemotherapy in HCC is multifactorial. HCC cells have overexpression of genes associated with drug resistance, such as MDR-1 and P-glycoprotein as well as high levels of dihydropyrimidine dehydrogenase. In addition, liver failure often necessitates dose reductions of potentially active drugs. Newer agents, such as gemcitabine and irinotecan, have not improved response rates.

Cisplatin-based combination chemotherapy regimens with interferon have been associated with improved response rates in advanced HCC. In one study, PIAF (cisplatin, interferon-α, doxorubicin, and infusional 5-FU) achieved a response in 13 of 50 patients (26%). Nine of those patients went on to surgical resection and four of those patients (44%) had no evidence of HCC on histological examination. A phase III trial comparing PIAF with single-agent doxorubicin is currently underway.

The present patient had recurrent hepatocellular carcinoma despite multiple local therapies. Because there is no standard systemic therapy for patients with advanced metastatic liver cancer, this man was treated on a clinical trial to explore the usefulness of a new biologic agent. Patients with advanced liver cancer should be considered as candidates for clinical trials of new biologics, drugs, or combinations of existing drugs, radiosensitizers, and radiation therapy. Palliation may sometimes be achieved in such studies.

Clinical Pearls

1. The incidence of hepatocellular carcinoma is on the rise in the United States and worldwide, likely due to the prevalence of hepatitis B and C.

2. Surgery is the only curative treatment for HCC.

3. An assessment of underlying liver function is critical for the purpose of determining the patient's ability to tolerate and benefit from therapy.

4. PIAF (cisplatin, interferon-α, doxorubicin, and infusional 5-FU) has shown promise in early studies, with response rates approximating 26%. A phase III trial is currently underway comparing PIAF to doxorubicin.

REFERENCES

1. Levy I, Sherman M; and Liver Cancer Study Group of the University of Toronto: Staging of hepatocellular carcinoma: Assessment of the CLIP, Okuda, and Child-Pugh staging systems in a cohort of 257 patients in Toronto. Gut 50:881-885, 2002.

2. El-Serag HB, Mason AC: Rising incidence of hepatocellular carcinoma in the United States. N Engl J Med 340(10):745-750, 1999.

3. Leung TW, Patt YZ, Lau WY, et al: Complete pathological remission is possible with systemic combination chemotherapy for inoperable hepatocellular carcinoma. Clin Cancer Res 5(7):1676-1681, 1999.

4. Poon RT, Fan ST, Lo CM, et al: Intrahepatic recurrence after curative resection of hepatocellular carcinoma: Long-term results of treatment and prognostic factors. Ann Surg 229(2):216-222, 1999.

5. Tagger A, Donato F, Ribero ML, et al: Case-control study on hepatitis C virus as a risk factor for hepatocellular carcinoma: The role of HCV genotypes and the synergism with hepatitis B virus and alcohol. Int J Cancer 81(5):695-699, 1999.

INDEX

Other Titles in the Pearls Series®

Duke	**Anesthesia Pearls**	1-56053-495-8
Carabello & Gazes	**Cardiology Pearls, 2nd Edition**	1-56053-403-6
Sahn & Heffner	**Critical Care Pearls, 2nd Edition**	1-56053-224-6
Sahn	**Dermatology Pearls**	1-56053-315-3
Baren & Alpern	**Emergency Medicine Pearls**	1-56053-575-X
Greenberg & Amato	**EMG Pearls**	1-56053-613-6
Jay	**Foot and Ankle Pearls**	1-56053-445-1
Concannon & Hurov	**Hand Pearls**	1-56053-463-X
Jones, King & Wofford	**Hypertension Pearls**	1-56053-583-0
Cunha	**Infectious Disease Pearls**	1-56053-203-3
Heffner & Sahn	**Internal Medicine Pearls, 2nd Edition**	1-56053-404-4
Mercado & Smetana	**Medical Consultation Pearls**	1-56053-504-0
Waclawik & Sutula	**Neurology Pearls**	1-56053-261-0
Gault	**Ophthalmology Pearls**	1-56053-498-2
Heffner & Byock	**Palliative and End-of-Life Pearls**	1-56053-500-8
Inselman	**Pediatric Pulmonary Pearls**	1-56053-350-1
Lennard	**Physical Medicine & Rehabilitation Pearls**	1-56053-455-9
Kolevzon & Stewart	**Psychiatry Pearls**	1-56053-590-3
Silver & Smith	**Rheumatology Pearls**	1-56053-201-7
Berry	**Sleep Medicine Pearls, 2nd Edition**	1-56053-490-7
Eck *et al.*	**Spine Pearls**	1-56053-571-7
Osterhoudt *et al.*	**Toxicology Pearls**	1-56053-614-4
Schluger & Harkin	**Tuberculosis Pearls**	1-56053-156-8
Resnick & Schaeffer	**Urology Pearls**	1-56053-351-X